Rheumatoid Arthritis
and *Proteus*

Alan Ebringer

Rheumatoid Arthritis and *Proteus*

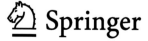 Springer

Alan Ebringer B.Sc., M.D.,
FRCP, FRACP, FRCPath
Professor of Immunology
King's College London and
Honorary Consultant
Rheumatologist
Middlesex Hospital
UCH School of Medicine
King's College London
Division of Life Sciences
Franklin-Wilkins Building
150 Stamford Street
London, SE1 8WA
UK

ISBN 978-0-85729-949-9   e-ISBN 978-0-85729-950-5
DOI 10.1007/978-0-85729-950-5
Springer London Dordrecht Heidelberg New York

British Library Cataloguing in Publication Data
A catalogue record for this book is available from the British Library

Library of Congress Control Number: 2011939310

Springer is part of Springer Science+Business Media (www.springer.com)

This book is dedicated to the memory of the late Dr. Mary Corbett (1933–2009) who was a Consultant Rheumatologist at the Middlesex Hospital (1969–1994) in London.

She was an excellent clinician, meticulous in her clinical care of patients and always available for friendly advice and support.

She was the first to start a "Rheumatoid Arthritis Prospective Study" (RAPS) in the UK which was a comprehensive and longitudinal investigation of the disease, and established that early treatment was necessary before erosive changes had occurred.

Mary Corbett was a co-author of the first paper which linked the urinary microbe Proteus to rheumatoid arthritis, the study having been carried out on her patients.

To my wife

Contents

Chapter 1
Scope and Distribution of the RA Problem

Contents

Rheumatoid Arthritis: An Introduction

Rheumatoid arthritis is a multi-system disorder characterised by chronic destructive synovitis attacking initially the small joints of the hands and feet but eventually producing generalised severe morbidity and an increased mortality.

There are over 20 million people in the world who suffer from this incapacitating disease, but the number of affected individuals may be higher if early stages or 'formes frustes' are included.

A. Ebringer, *Rheumatoid Arthritis and Proteus*,
DOI 10.1007/978-0-85729-950-5_1,
© Springer-Verlag London Limited 2012

The disease is not only a health problem for the affected individual but is also a social burden to society in the costs involved in caring and treating such patients.

Extensive research studies have been carried out over the last 100 years to try and characterise the onset and cause of this disease.

Predisposing genetic factors have been discovered over the last 30 years which could throw some light on the origin of this debilitating condition.

Clinical Features of Rheumatoid Arthritis

The onset of the disease is often insidious, and the patient may complain of transient muscular pains, stiffness, tiredness, malaise, and fatigue before any joint symptoms appear.

Some patients present with acute episodes of pain involving, in the typical case, the small joints of the fingers and toes which are usually the first ones to become involved.

Swelling of the proximal interphalangeal joints gives rise to the typical spindled appearance of the fingers.

As the disease progresses, it involves the wrists, elbows, shoulders, ankles and knees. Muscular stiffness is a prominent symptom, especially in the mornings or after periods of inactivity.

The joints become swollen and painful due to a proliferative synovial response characterised by cellular hyperplasia, pannus formation, increased vascularity and release of hydrolytic enzymes and interleukins which lead to progressive destruction of cartilage, ligaments and bone.

A key role in pathological damage is caused by TNF-α (Brennan et al. 1992). Metalloproteinases secreted by inflammatory synovial fibroblasts cause cartilage destruction which leads to further physical disability (Aletaha et al. 2011).

Characteristic subcutaneous rheumatoid nodules may appear on the ulnar aspect of the forearm and other points of pressure in about 10% of rheumatoid arthritis patients.

During active phases of the disease, a low-grade fever may be present with a normocytic anaemia and an elevated erythrocyte sedimentation rate. As the disease advances, muscle spasms give rise to flexion deformities in the joints. Later permanent and irreversible contractures develop, the joints become completely disorganised and not amenable to surgery. A characteristic deformity in the hands is anterior subluxation of the metacarpophalangeal joints and ulnar deviation of the fingers.

In the early stages, radiographic examination shows only bony demineralization, but later the joint space becomes narrower and marginal erosions appear.

The extra-articular manifestations may involve a diffuse vasculitis, with leg ulcers, episcleritis, keratoconjunctivitis sicca, scleromalacia perforans, pericarditis, pleurisy and peripheral neuropathy.

The disease progressively leads to widespread muscular atrophy, fibrous or bony ankylosis, and radiological examination may show osteoarthrosis.

The Disability of Rheumatoid Arthritis

Rheumatoid arthritis, as it progresses, is an extremely disabling and debilitating disease. Hand deformities lead to gradual loss of function, the patient cannot open doors, drive a car, hold a spoon or go to the toilet without encountering serious difficulties in daily living.

In the Calderdale study, 67% of rheumatoid arthritis patients reported that the disease limited their daily activity, 60% said that it affected their ability to lead a normal life and 50% were always in pain (Badley and Tennant 1993).

The prevalence of rheumatoid arthritis increases with age in both men and women, and since there is a demographic growth in Western societies of individuals aged over 60 years, this suggests the rheumatoid arthritis–associated morbidity, mortality and disability are likely to increase among older adults in the future (Helmick et al. 2008).

The Social and Financial Costs of Rheumatoid Arthritis

Rheumatoid arthritis is a musculo-skeletal disorder with a high prevalence throughout the developed world having a clinical course which progressively degrades the patient's quality of life and reduces his or her life expectancy.

The annual cost of rheumatoid arthritis has been estimated to be between one and two billion pounds in the UK (McIntosh 1996).

Similar American studies have shown that annual costs of rheumatoid arthritis, through hospital costs, loss of income and carer expenditure amount to well over ten billion dollars (Yelin 1996).

A related large study from Madrid showed that the annual economic impact of rheumatoid arthritis to the Spanish society might be more than two billion American dollars which clearly highlights the substantial burden that this disease imposes on modern society (Lajas et al. 2003).

The therapy of rheumatoid arthritis involves not only the use of non-steroidal anti-inflammatory drugs, methotrexate, sometimes steroids but also newer biological preparations which place an exorbitant financial strain on health providers and society in general. Many of these drugs have undesirable side effects.

The general principle in such a therapy is to reduce the intensity of the inflammation once it has started in a patient.

Inflammation is the body's response to injury. The question arises 'What has been responsible for the tissue injury?', in other words what is the primary cause which sets off rheumatoid arthritis.

A possible way as to how to answer such a question may be to look for previous successful solutions in finding the cause of a disease and no better example is provided than by rheumatic fever.

Molecular Mimicry and Rheumatic Fever

The prototype of an autoimmune disease evoked by an external agent and operating through the mechanism of 'molecular mimicry' is rheumatic fever.

It usually occurs some 2–4 weeks after an upper respiratory tract infection by Lancefield group A *Streptococci*. Some *Streptococci* have been found to have antigens which crossreact with cardiac myosin and others resemble some molecular sequences found in the basal ganglia of the brain. When someone develops tonsillitis by this microbe, the resultant antibodies will not only attack the *Streptococcal* bacteria but also the heart and the brain. Thus, anti-*Streptococcal* antibodies produce rheumatic fever and Sydenham's chorea by acting as cytopathic autoantibodies. It would appear that rheumatic fever and Sydenham's chorea are autoimmune diseases caused by an infection.

Other diseases operate by a similar mechanism. Some 20–30 million individuals in South America, especially Brazil, are infected by the protozoan parasite *Trypanosoma cruzi*. Patients with Chaga's disease have antibodies which react with both antigens present on the surface of the parasite as well as with cardiac endothelium and myocardium, giving rise to a myocarditis which pathologically resembles rheumatic fever. Thus, it would appear that even parasites can be triggers or causative agents of an autoimmune disease (Ebringer et al. 2003).

It is not inconceivable that a similar mechanism may operate in rheumatoid arthritis.

The Properties of the Rheumatoid Arthritis Problem

To investigate a 'scientific problem', it is relevant to note the properties of the problem which define the puzzle or question. It is these properties that provide possible answers for the scientific enquiry. The philosopher of science Karl Popper has always emphasised that in trying to solve a scientific problem, one must generate hypotheses which can then be tested experimentally. For such hypotheses to be labelled as scientific, they must prohibit certain results. If such prohibited results are obtained, then the theory is found to be invalid or has failed in explaining the 'scientific problem'. We then must produce new hypotheses to tackle the problem under investigation. So scientific research proceeds by a succession of conjectures or guesses and refutations.

The properties of the rheumatoid arthritis problem would appear to be the following:

1. *Sex ratio*: Rheumatoid arthritis is found three to four times more frequently in women than men.
2. *Smokers*: Rheumatoid arthritis is found more frequently in smokers than non-smokers (Klareskog et al. 2007). However, smokers suffer more from urinary tract infections than non-smokers.
3. *Post-puerperal onset*: Rheumatoid arthritis often starts 3–6 weeks after the end of a pregnancy. However, urinary tract infections also occur frequently during and after a pregnancy.
4. *Identical twin studies*: Rheumatoid arthritis is not found very frequently in the second identical twin when the first twin has the disease. Several studies have been published which indicate a low 'concordance rate': Finland 12% (Aho et al. 1986), England 15% (Silman et al. 1993), and Denmark 10% (Svendsen et al. 2002). These identical twin studies suggest that there is an environmental factor associated with the onset of rheumatoid arthritis.
5. *Genetic links*: Rheumatoid arthritis is found more frequently in individuals belonging to HLA-DR4 (Stastny et al. 1988) and HLA-DR1 (Schiff et al. 1982) groups. Over 90% of rheumatoid arthritis patients belong to the HLA-DR1/4 groups whilst the frequency of these groups in the general population is about 35%.

It is proposed to use these properties of the rheumatoid arthritis problem to investigate the possible cause of this disease by research workers associated with the King's College Immunology Unit in London.

King's College Immunology Unit

The Women's Department of King's College London opened in 1885 and in 1915 moved to Campden Hill road, Kensington.

In 1953, it received a Royal Charter and was named Queen Elizabeth College after the Queen Mother.

The college distinguished itself in teaching and research in microbiology, biochemistry, physiology and nutrition. In 1972, an Immunology Unit was set up within the departments of biochemistry and microbiology with an interest in research into genetic and environmental factors in rheumatic diseases, especially ankylosing spondylitis and rheumatoid arthritis. Many students and doctoral candidates passed through the Unit and two stayed for over 20 years, Dr. Clyde Wilson Ph.D., MRCPath and Dr. Taha Rashid MBChB, M.Phil.

In 1985, Queen Elizabeth College remerged with King's College and moved to the Waterloo Campus in Stamford street on the South Bank.

Rheumatoid arthritis has been a research interest of the Unit since 1978 when Professor Stastny from Dallas showed that the disease was linked to the Major Histocompatibility antigen HLA-DR4 (Stastny 1978).

A leading American research worker has stated that the chronic inflammatory reaction in the rheumatoid synovial membrane is the result of an active immune response (Ziff et al. 1988). It is the aim of this book to try and identify the origin of such an immune response.

References

Aho K, Koskenvuo M, Tuominen J, Kaprio J. Occurrence of rheumatoid arthritis in a nationwide series of twins. J Rheumatol. 1986;13: 899–902.

Aletaha D, Funovits J, Smolen JS. Physical disability in rheumatoid arthritis is associated with cartilage damage rather than bone destruction. Ann Rheum Dis. 2011;70:733–9.

Badley EM, Tennant A. Impact of disablement due to rheumatic disorders in a British population: estimates of severity and prevalence from the Calderdale Rheumatic Disablement Survey. Ann Rheum Dis. 1993;52:6–13.

Brennan FM, Maini RN, Feldmann M. TNF-α – a pivotal role in rheumatoid arthritis? Br J Rheumatol. 1992;31:293–8.

Ebringer A, Rashid T, Wilson C. Molecular mimicry as the basis of new theory of autoimmunity. In: Zouali M, editor. Frontiers in autoimmunity. Amsterdam/Washington, DC: IOS Press; 2003. p. 79–99.

Helmick CG, Felson DT, Lawrence RC, Gabriel S, Hirsch R, Kwoh CK, et al. Estimates of prevalence of arthritis and other rheumatic conditions in the United States. Arthritis Rheum. 2008;58:15–25.

Klareskog L, Padyukov L, Alfredsson L. Smoking as a trigger for inflammatory rheumatic diseases. Curr Opin Rheumatol. 2007;A 19:49–54.

Lajas C, Abasolo L, Belladel B, Hernadez-Garcia C, Carmona L, Vargas E, et al. Costs and predictors of costs in rheumatoid arthritis: a prevalence based study. Arthritis Rheum. 2003;49:64–70.

McIntosh E. The costs of rheumatoid arthritis. Br J Rheumatol. 1996;35:781–90.

Schiff B, Mizrachi Y, Orgad S, Yaron M, Gazit E. Association of HLA-Aw 31 and HLA-DR1 with adult rheumatoid arthritis. Ann Rheum Dis. 1982;41:403–4.

Silman AJ, MacGregor AJ, Thomson W, Holligan S, Carthy D, Farhan A, et al. Twin concordance rates for rheumatoid arthritis: results from a nationwide study. Br J Rheumatol. 1993;32:903–7.

Stastny P. Association of the B-cell alloantigen DRw4 with rheumatoid arthritis. New Engl J Med. 1978;298:869–71.

Stastny P, Ball EJ, Khan MA, Olsen NJ, Pincus T, Gao X. HLA-DR4 and other genetic markers in rheumatoid arthritis. Br J Rheumatol. 1988;27(Suppl II):132–8.

Svendsen AJ, Holm NV, Kyvik K, Petersen PH, Junker P. Relative importance of genetic effects in rheumatoid arthritis: historical cohort study of Danish nationwide twin population. Br Med J. 2002;324:264–6.

Yelin EK. The cost of rheumatoid arthritis; absolute, incremental and marginal estimates. J Rheumatol. 1996;23:47–51.

Ziff M, Cavender D, Haskard D. Pathogenetic factors in rheumatoid synovitis. Br J Rheumatol. 1988;27(Suppl II):153–6.

Chapter 2
History of the Attempts to Find the Cause of RA

Contents

Introduction

There has been a continuous debate about the origin and early detection of rheumatoid arthritis. The strongest evidence suggesting recent onset is the absence of the disease in Egyptian mummies. Other rheumatological diseases such as

A. Ebringer, *Rheumatoid Arthritis and Proteus*,
DOI 10.1007/978-0-85729-950-5_2,
© Springer-Verlag London Limited 2012

osteoarthritis, ankylosing spondylitis, gout and chondrocalcinosis are well represented in Egyptian bone specimens and this appeared to be convincing evidence to Professor Watson Buchanan from Glasgow that rheumatoid arthritis was a disease of recent onset which appeared in the last two centuries (Buchanan and Kean 2001).

The presence of erosions in specimens from palaeolithic, antique and medieval cemeteries has been hotly disputed as being due to chemical conditions in the soil and not representing evidence of rheumatoid arthritis.

Another suggestion has been that increased milk consumption occurred during the nineteenth and twentieth centuries, and this has been somehow involved in the onset of rheumatoid arthritis. A similar suggestion has been proposed that type I diabetes correlates well with increased consumption of milk in many countries.

There are two names that dominate the debate about the origin and definition of rheumatoid arthritis. One is that of Landré-Beauvais from Paris and the other one is that of Alfred Baring Garrod from London. They provide a convenient framework to divide the investigations into the origin of rheumatoid arthritis.

The phase before Landré-Beauvais consists of various descriptions which could or could not be called cases of rheumatoid arthritis, involving Roman, Byzantine and Mexican sources.

There has also been an exhaustive investigations of paintings, especially from Dutch and Flemish masters asking whether spindling of fingers was an accurate and realistic portrayal of the sitter or a stylistic exaggeration of post-Renaissance Mannerism (Dequeker 1977).

After Landré-Beauvais, there is an inter-regnum or a period of some 60 years where clinical descriptions appear to resemble modern descriptions of rheumatoid arthritis.

Finally with Alfred Baring Garrod who coined the word 'rheumatoid arthritis', we reach modern times and the search for the cause of this disease.

Rheumatoid Arthritis in Antiquity, India and Byzantium

Examination of burial sites provides a useful way of assessing the distribution of arthritic lesions in a population. The pattern of arthritis in Roman Britain was investigated by examining the skeletons of 416 adults from the Roman cemetery at Poundbury Camp near Dorchester in Dorset (Thould and Thould 1983).

When the Romans invaded Britain in A.D. 43, they soon subjugated the southern Celtic kingdoms. The legion Augusta II, under the command of the future emperor Vespasian, defeated the Celtic Durotriges in a fierce battle at Maiden Castle in Dorset. Around A.D. 70, Durnovaria, which is nowadays known as Dorchester, was built with a forum, public baths, shops, running water and fine houses. Over the next four centuries, the dead were buried in the large Roman cemetery at Poundbury outside the walls. The majority of the inhabitants were Celts being descendants of the Belgae who emigrated to Britain around 100 B.C. They were farmers, artisans and led a physically hard life with a life expectancy of about 40 years. In the 416 skeletons examined, there was a high prevalence of osteoarthritis with particularly severe changes in the vertebral column.

Inflammatory joint disease was seen in two examples. The first was a man with severe inflammatory and exuberant new bone formation affecting the two metacarpo-phalangeal joints and two proximal inter-phalangeal joints in the hands. Radiographic examination showed erosions in the carpus.

The other example was in a woman where inflammatory changes were seen affecting one knee joint, both wrist joints and the right elbow joint. There was fusion of the bones of one foot, including the first and fifth tarsal metatarsal joints. The radiographs of the hands showed erosions of the carpus and metacarpals. The appearances in both of these subjects were compatible with a diagnosis of rheumatoid arthritis.

The finding of two skeletons showing rheumatoid arthritis in a Roman-Celtic population would tend to suggest that it is not a disease of recent onset. The Thoulds argue that 'if we assume the prevalence was about 0.5%, rather than the current British population of 1–2% overall, we would expect to find two examples in a collection 416 skeletons, which was indeed what we found. We contend therefore that rheumatoid arthritis is as old as historical man'.

The oldest proposed written account of a disease that could be called 'rheumatoid arthritis' is generally ascribed to Scribonius Largus who was a military physician and accompanied Julius Caesar on some of his campaigns. Scribonius Largus wrote about a polyarthritis occurring mainly in elderly women. A Roman woman was considered elder between the ages of 35 and 45 years because the general life expectancy was around 40 years.

There is also evidence of the presence of a chronic symmetric polyarthritis in the 'Karaka Samhita', a medical text from India written between 500 B.C. and 100 A.D. The patients had subcutaneous nodules, contractures and sometimes atrophy of the limbs.

A Byzantine emperor, Monomachus Constantine IX (A.D. 980–1055), seems to have been the first illustrious sufferer from rheumatoid arthritis (Caughey 1974). A description of his disease is given by Michael Psellus in his book 'Chronographia' where he describes the emperor suffering recurrent polyarthritis, deformities of the hands and subsequent disability. Professor Watson Buchanan comments 'with delight to us Scottish Presbyterians that according to Psellus, the emperor was naturally inclined to sexual indulgence but could find no satisfaction in cheap harlotry'.

Rheumatoid Arthritis in Mexico

In an examination of the skeletal remains kept at the National Museum of Anthropology of Mexico, 21 cases of erosive arthritis have been studied; 8 skeletons of the Preclassical era (Tlatilco 1400–600 B.C.), 5 of the Classic era

(Teotihuacan 200 B.C. to 600 A.D.) and 8 from the Post-classic era (A.D. 800–1500). Erosions were found on the articular surfaces, the edges of the articular surfaces and at the capsular insertions of carpal, metacarpo-phalangeal, tarsal and metatarso-phalangeal joints. These appearances were similar to those seen in patients with rheumatoid arthritis (Aceves-Avila et al. 2001).

In 1578, Alonso Lopez de Hinojosos, working in the Hospital Real de San José de los Naturales, in Mexico City, described two different types of gout, one classical gout with tophi as hard nodules and a second type which was a chronic condition of the same joints and disabled the patients by severe contractures and muscular atrophy (Aceves-Avila et al. 2002).

Thomas Sydenham (1624–1689) also distinguished gout from another chronic arthritis resembling rheumatoid arthritis but had been preceded in this description by Lopez de Hinojosos by some 100 years. One of Sydenham's patients also had swan-neck deformities of the fingers.

Evidence from Paintings

In the 'Temptation of Saint Anthony' now in the Escorial Palace near Madrid, a beggar is shown with hand and wrist deformities which resemble those found in patients with rheumatoid arthritis whilst no such deformities can be seen in the other portrayed individuals.

The 'Birth of Venus', now in the Uffizi Gallery in Florence, was painted in 1486 by Sandro Botticelli (1445–1510) and shows characteristic swellings of the proximal inter-phalangeal joints of the right hand suggestive of rheumatoid arthritis. The model for the painting was a married noblewoman Simonetta Vespucci, it is said almost his muse, and Botticelli asked to be buried near her, in the Chiesa di Ognissanti in Florence after his death.

The man in the painting of 'The Donators' by Jan Gossaert also known as Mabuse (1478–1532) has polyarthritis of the fingers of his left hand with flexion deformities of the second, fourth and fifth fingers, suggestive of rheumatoid arthritis.

In the 'Painter's family' by Jacobo Jordaen (1593–1678), the hands of the serving maid show symmetrical inflammation of the metacarpo-phalangeal joints which are not seen in three other individuals in the painting.

In several paintings by Peter Paul Rubens (1577–1640), hand deformities characteristic of rheumatoid arthritis are clearly depicted.

The painter Siebrandus Sixtius (1538–1631) produced two portraits in which the hands reveal swelling of metacarpo-phalangeal and proximal inter-phalangeal joints, with ulnar deviations and flexion contractures of the fingers (Dequeker 1992).

Landré-Beauvais at the Salpêtrière in Paris

The first unequivocal description of rheumatoid arthritis was made by Augustin Jacob Landré-Beauvais (1772–1840) in Paris. He was born in Orléans and studied under Pierre Joseph Desault and Marie François Xavier Bichat in Paris. From 1772, he pursued his medical education under Jean Louis Petit in Lyon.

In 1796, he obtained an internship at the Salpêtrière, even then a famous hospital where he assisted Philippe Pinel. In 1799, he was appointed professor of clinical medicine at the Salpêtrière which is located on the rive gauche next to the Jardin des Plantes. After the restoration, he also held a chair of medicine at the Paris Polytechnic School. He was removed in 1830 from this post at the insistence of King Louis-Philippe of France.

He proposed and defended his Medical Thesis at the École de Médicine which is situated on the Boulevard Saint Germain in the Latin Quarter on the 16th Thermidor of the year VIII (3rd August 1800).

The ponderous and provocative title of his thesis was 'Doit-on admettre une nouvelle espèce de goutte sous la dénomination de goutte asthénique primitive?'. The rough translation would be 'Should we accept a new type of gout, under the name of primary debilitating gout?'

Landré-Beauvais described a new syndrome on the basis of nine long-term female residents of the Salpêtrière. He clearly points out the new disease can be distinguished from classical gout. He says the condition occurs mostly in women, with characteristic capsular swelling, limitation of motion of the joints in the hands and fingers and may spread to other joints. Over time, there is the development of bony ankylosis with disorganisation of many joints (Snorrason 1952).

He was emphatic in his view that this was a new clinical condition or syndrome although he was not clear whether it was linked to gout. This new nosological concept was considered by the late Professor Eric Bywaters from the Postgraduate Medical School at the Hammersmith Hospital, a doyen of British rheumatology as the 'first sighting of the disease' (Bywaters 1988).

Alfred Baring Garrod at University College and King's College Hospitals in London

Alfred Baring Garrod was born in Ipswich. He was initially apprenticed at Ipswich Hospital but later moved to University College Hospital in London.

In 1859, he coined the name of 'rheumatoid arthritis' and clearly distinguished it from gout.

In 1863, he became Professor of Materia Medica and Therapeutics at King's College Hospital.

He had an extensive private practice and lived on premises at 63 Harley street, in London.

There is a street in the balneal town of Aix-les-Bains named after him.

In 1890, he was knighted and appointed 'Physician Extraordinary' to Queen Victoria (Fig. 2.1).

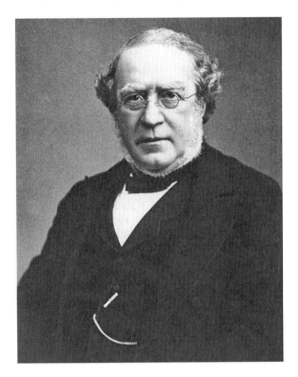

FIGURE 2.1 Photograph of Sir Alfred Baring Garrod who coined the term 'rheumatoid arthritis' (With kind permission from the Wellcome Library, London)

Bacteriological Theory

Following the microbial discoveries of Louis Pasteur and Robert Koch, the possibility of infection by microbes crept into the virgin field of rheumatology.

One of the first to recognize the possibility of germs as the cause of the disease was Thomas Maclagen who in 1876 introduced salicin for the treatment of rheumatic fever.

In 1901, William Hunter in London inaugurated the idea of 'focal sepsis' which was a bonanza for dentists, otorhinolaryngologists and even general surgeons who began to strip rheumatoid arthritis patients of their teeth, adenoids, tonsils, appendices, gall bladders and even their colons. In the United States, this was exploited on a large scale by Frank Billings in Chicago and by Ed Rosenow at the Mayo Clinic.

Virology Versus Bacteriology

A variety of viral agents have been suggested as causing direct infections of joints and thereby causing rheumatoid arthritis: Epstein–Barr virus, human parvovirus B19 and rubella.

Epstein–Barr virus would appear to be a likely candidate; however, there are some problems with this hypothesis. Epstein–Barr virus establishes persistent infection in 90% of individuals within the first years of life.

Rheumatoid arthritis is a disease predominantly of middle-aged females whilst Epstein–Barr virus exposure occurs in children aged less than 5 years. It is the wrong time-frame.

Clinical and animal studies have suggested a role for parvovirus B19 to be involved, but this could not be confirmed by other workers.

A similar lack of evidence applies to rubella, mumps and measles viruses which are diseases of concern mainly to paediatric physicians.

Other bacterial suggestions have been mycobacteria or mycoplasmas but again with no permanent convincing evidence (Rashid and Ebringer 2007).

Conclusions

Although sightings of clinical conditions resembling rheumatoid arthritis have been made throughout history, it is possible that the low life expectancy of 40 years may have precluded the florid and numerous cases of the condition we find in modern times. Increased life expectancy produced by knowledge of microbes, adequate sewage disposal, general hygiene, good nutrition, general use of antibiotics and better scientific theories of disease has resulted in a different medical scene compared to the one seen by medical practitioners of old.

The revolutionary definition of new syndromes or diseases as described by Landré-Beauvais and Garrod has produced a recognition of clinical phenomena which may have been around for a long time but was not present in extant medical textbooks and therefore was not condoned by the medical establishments. It is to their credit that they recognised novel forms of disease in their patients.

In view of numerous probable sightings throughout history, it is unlikely that rheumatoid arthritis could be considered as a disease originating in the last 200 years. If a urinary microbe is involved, then the 'theory of recent onset of rheumatoid arthritis' may require some revision.

References

Aceves-Avila FJ, Medina F, Fraga A. The antiquity of rheumatoid arthritis: a reappraisal. J Rheumatol. 2001;28:751–7.

Aceves-Avila FJ, Delgadillo-Ruano MA, Ramos-Remus C, Gomez-Vargas A. The "Hospital Real de San Josef de Los Naturales" and the rheumatic conditions found in New Spain during the sixteenth century. Reumatismo. 2002;54:62–6.

Buchanan WW, Kean WE. Rheumatoid arthritis: beyond the lymphocyte. J Rheumatol. 2001;28:691–2.

Bywaters E. Historical aspects of the aetiology of rheumatoid arthritis. Br J Rheumatol. 1988;27 Suppl 2:110–5.

Caughey DE. The arthritis of Constantine IX. Ann Rheum Dis. 1974;33:77–80.

Dequeker J. Arthritis in Flemish paintings. Br Med J. 1977;1:1203–5.

Dequeker J. Siebrandus Sixtius: evidence of rheumatoid arthritis of the robust reaction type in a seventeenth century priest. Ann Rheum Dis. 1992;51:561–2.

Rashid T, Ebringer A. Rheumatoid arthritis is linked to Proteus – the evidence. Clin Rheumatol. 2007;26:1036–43.

Snorrason E. Landré-Beauvais and his "Goutte Asthénique Primitive." ACTA Med SCAND. 1952; 142, Suppl. 266:115–8.

Thould AK, Thould BT. Arthritis in Roman Britain. Br Med J. 1983; 287:1909–11.

Chapter 3
HLA-DR1/4 and Antibodies to *Proteus* in London

Contents

The Middlesex Hospital in London

The first Middlesex Hospital opened in 1745 as the Middlesex Infirmary in Windmill street London W1. The second Middlesex Hospital opened in 1757 in Mortimer street and

A. Ebringer, *Rheumatoid Arthritis and Proteus*,
DOI 10.1007/978-0-85729-950-5_3,
© Springer-Verlag London Limited 2012

was incorporated by an Act of Parliament in 1836. The new building was opened in 1935, by the Duke of York, later to become King George VI.

The hospital lobby contained four large paintings, entitled 'Acts of Mercy' by Frederick Cayley Robinson, completed in 1920. After the merger of the Middlesex Hospital with University College Hospital in 1994, the paintings were acquired by the Wellcome Collection.

The Middlesex Hospital was where Dr. WSC 'Will' Copeman had his early appointment as Senior Consultant in Rheumatology in the Arthur Stanley Institute before he wrote his 'Textbook of Rheumatic Diseases'.

Professor Eric Bywaters, the doyen of academic rheumatologists, graduated from the Middlesex Hospital.

The post-war services in rheumatology were provided by Dr. Oswald Savage. The Department of Rheumatology at the Middlesex Hospital was founded by Dr. Archibald Cabbourn Boyle, known as 'Bill' and was located in Arthur Stanley House, after it merged with the Arthur Stanley Institute, in Tottenham street, next to the main hospital.

Arthur Stanley House was opened by Her Majesty the Queen in 1965 and became a centre dedicated to the care of rheumatic patients.

The building also contained a physiotherapy and rehabilitation section as well as a Department of Immunology, under Professor Ivan Roitt.

Bill Boyle was a gifted teacher, and by the time of his retirement he had had a hand in training one third of the rheumatologists in the UK and many from overseas, especially Australasia.

Dr. Mary Corbett was appointed as a second Consultant in Rheumatology and started longitudinal studies on rheumatoid arthritis, known as 'Rheumatoid Arthritis Prospective Studies' or RAPS for short.

She emphasised that early treatment was paramount to prevent the development of irreversible bony changes and deformities. She approved the studies on antibodies to *Proteus* which were carried out on her rheumatoid arthritis patients attending the weekly 'Gold Clinic'.

Professor David Isenberg was appointed Professor of Rheumatology for the merged Middlesex University College Hospitals and collaborated in some studies in both ankylosing spondylitis and rheumatoid arthritis patients carried out by the King's College group. Dr. Michael Shipley was appointed Consultant in Rheumatology and provided clinical advice for the 'Ankylosing Spondylitis Research Clinic' and support in running two International Symposia held at the Middlesex Hospital in 1983 and 1987. Professor Jonathan Edwards contributed to the international symposia and showed that chemical ablation of B cells led to improvement in patients with rheumatoid arthritis.

The 'Ankylosing Spondylitis Research Clinic of the Middlesex Hospital'

In 1973, two seminal observations were published one from the Westminster Hospital in London and the other one from Terasaki's group in Los Angeles, that over 95% of patients with ankylosing spondylitis carried the major histocompatibility marker, HLA-B27, whilst it was present in only 8% of the general population. Clearly, here was a puzzle that required some form of explanation.

Dr. D.C.O. James, the immunologist involved in the discovery of HLA-B27 at the Westminster Hospital, came to the immunology lectures at Queen Elizabeth College, now part of King's College, and discussed this problem.

The suggestion from our group was that there was probably some form of 'molecular mimicry' between an unknown microbe and HLA-B27.

This was based on the precedent of rheumatic fever and Sydenham's chorea being caused by anti-*streptococcal* antibodies following an upper respiratory tract infection such as tonsillitis.

It was decided to study this question and Dr. Bill Boyle was approached with the suggestion that this could be investigated in an 'Ankylosing Spondylitis Research Clinic'. He gave his approval and supported the clinic with financial resources. The clinic was started by my brother, Dr. Roland Ebringer who was in charge of the clinical studies till 1980 when he returned to Australia.

The immunological studies were carried out at Queen Elizabeth College and the clinical studies at the Middlesex Hospital. Some 900 ankylosing spondylitis patients were seen at the clinic between 1975 and 2002 when the clinic was closed.

In 1975, molecular mimicry was demonstrated between the bowel microbe *Klebsiella* and HLA-B27. Faecal studies showed that *Klebsiella* microbes could be isolated from active ankylosing spondylitis patients and later elevated levels of antibodies to *Klebsiella* could be demonstrated by several techniques.

When 2 years later, Professor Stastny from Dallas showed that rheumatoid arthritis patients were found more frequently in carriers of HLA-DR4; it was considered that the same explanation might apply to this observation as it did for *Streptococcus* and rheumatic fever or *Klebsiella* and ankylosing spondylitis.

Dr. Mary Corbett gave her approval that her rheumatoid arthritis patients could be investigated by the same methods as the patients in the 'Ankylosing Spondylitis Research Clinic'.

Investigation into a Possible Link Between HLA-DR4 and Bacteria

Serum was obtained from a rabbit prior to immunisation to be used as a control sample. Then the rabbit was immunised with 'Ficoll'-separated lymphocytes from two 40-ml samples of venous blood obtained from a patient with severe rheumatoid arthritis, whose HLA-DR tissue type was DR4,X and who was rheumatoid factor–positive. Rabbit serum taken before and after four immunisations was tested by immunodiffusion against soluble extracts from 18 different bacteria.

TABLE 3.1 Microorganisms used in immunodiffusion studies

Microorganism	Culture reference number
Gram-negative bacteria	
Enterobacter cloacae	QEC B27
Shigella sonnei	QEC B21
Salmonella typhimurium	QEC B22
Escherichia coli	QEC B35
Pseudomonas aeruginosa	QEC B15
Proteus vulgaris	QEC B11
Proteus mirabilis	QEC B17
Alcaligenes faecalis	QEC B18
Gram-positive bacteria	
Bacillus subtilis	QEC S6
Streptococcus faecalis	QEC D2
Streptococcus pyogenes	QEC D10
Streptococcus viridans	QEC D15
Streptococcus lactis	QEC D8
Staphylococcus albus	QEC C1
Staphylococcus aureus	QEC C22
Staphylococcus aureus	St. Stephen's.
Streptococcus pyogenes	St. Stephen's
Streptococcus pneumoniae	St. Stephen's
Yeast	
Candida albicans	St. Stephen's

QEC Queen Elizabeth College collection, St. Stephen's Hospital

Microorganisms were obtained from the Microbiology Department at Queen Elizabeth College and from the Department of Microbiology at St. Stephen's Hospital (Table 3.1).

Gram-positive and gram-negative bacteria were plated on blood and MacConkey agar, incubated at 37°C for 18 h. Individual colonies were subcultured and incubated at 37°C for a further 48 h.

Pure bacterial broth cultures were centrifuged, washed three times with phosphate-buffered saline (pH 7.4) containing 0.08% sodium azide, resuspended, and ultrasonicated. The supernatants were used as antigen solutions for immunodiffusion studies.

Immunodiffusion plates containing 1% agar (Oxoid) and 0.1% sodium azide were prepared to a depth of 1 cm, a centre well and four peripheral wells, each 5 mm from the centre well were cut. Rabbit serum was placed in the centre well and bacterial or yeast sonicates in the peripheral wells.

The rabbit antiserum gave five precipitin lines against *Enterobacter cloacae*, *Salmonella typhimurium*, *Alcaligenes faecalis*, as well as against *Proteus mirabilis* and *Proteus vulgaris*. However, the pre-immunisation serum also produced precipitin lines against the first three microbial sonicates, namely *Enterobacter cloacae*, *Salmonella typhimurium* and *Alcaligenes faecalis*.

However, the interesting observation was that the HLA-DR4-immunised rabbit serum produced precipitin lines against *Proteus* bacteria, microorganisms which are the second commonest cause of urinary tract infections, especially in the upper urinary tract. It became apparent that a urinary tract infection could readily explain the preponderance of rheumatoid arthritis in women.

Proteus bacteria are ubiquitous in nature: They are found in soil, on vegetables, in water, sewage, mammalian gut and vagina.

These bacteria have also been incriminated in opportunistic infections especially in wounds, burns, throat and ear infections as well as in bronchitis and chest infections.

The suggestion arises that *Proteus* bacteria may be involved in this disease, and if this hypothesis is correct, then antibodies to this microbe should be demonstrable in rheumatoid arthritis patients.

Patients and Controls

Sera from Rheumatoid Arthritis Patients

Serum samples were obtained from 30 rheumatoid arthritis patients attending the weekly 'Gold Clinic' at the Middlesex Hospital.

It was considered that rheumatoid arthritis requiring second-line therapy represented a group with more active disease than rheumatoid arthritis patients being treated with non-steroidal anti-inflammatory drugs.

There were 14 male and 16 women. Their mean age was 59 years (Range: 40–78 years) and the diagnosis was made according to the American Rheumatism Association criteria (Ropes et al. 1958).

All serum samples were investigated for C-reactive protein, IgG and IgA by the single radial immunodiffusion method of Mancini.

The hospital service measured the erythrocyte sedimentation rate (ESR) of all patients by the method of Westergren.

The mean (± standard error) erythrocyte sedimentation rate (ESR) in the rheumatoid arthritis was 28.2 ± 5.2 mm/h and the mean (± standard error) C-reactive protein level was 22.7 ± 5.6 µg/ml (Table 3.2).

Sera from Ankylosing Spondylitis Patients

Serum samples were obtained from 52 patients with ankylosing spondylitis, satisfying the New York criteria (Bennet and Wood 1968) and attending the 'Ankylosing Spondylitis Research Clinic' of the Middlesex Hospital.

Ankylosing spondylitis patients with serum IgA greater or equal to 3 g/l were allocated to the active ankylosing spondylitis group and those with serum IgA less than 3 g/l and erythrocyte sedimentation rate less than 15 mm/h were placed in the inactive group. Ankylosing spondylitis patients with a serum IgA less than 3 g/l but with an erythrocyte sedimentation rate

TABLE 3.2 Characteristics of the study groups

	Controls	Active AS	Inactive AS	RA
Number	41	24	28	30
M/F	23/18	20/4	21/7	14/16
Age range	20–50	28–62	24–69	40–78
Mean age	ND	41	44	59
ESR mm/h	ND	41.6 ± 5.0	5.7 ± 1.0	28.2 ± 5.2
CRP µg/ml	1.6 ± 0.6	35.9 ± 5.8	3.8 ± 0.8	22.7 ± 5.6
IgG g/l	12.4 ± 0.4	20.6 ± 0.1	14.0 ± 0.8	15.2 ± 0.9
IgA g/l	1.96 ± 0.1	4.74 ± 0.2	1.74 ± 0.1	2.55 ± 0.2

AS ankylosing spondylitis, *RA* rheumatoid arthritis, *ESR* erythrocyte sedimentation rate, *CRP* C-reactive protein, *ND* Not done, Mean ± standard error, *M/F* Male/Female, Mean age: years

above 15 mm/h were excluded from the study. Previous studies had shown that active ankylosing spondylitis patients had elevated levels of serum IgA (Cowling et al. 1980).

Control sera were samples obtained from 41 healthy blood donors.

Statistical Analysis of Patient Groups and Controls

The mean (± standard error) erythrocyte sedimentation rate in the rheumatoid arthritis group was 28.2 ± 5.2 mm/h and this was significantly higher ($p < 0.001$, $t = 4.17$) than the level of 5.7 ± 1.0 mm/h found in the inactive ankylosing spondylitis group.

The mean (± standard error) erythrocyte sedimentation rate in the active ankylosing spondylitis was 41.6 ± 5.0 mm/h and this was significantly higher ($p < 0.001$, $t = 7.67$) than the level of 5.7 ± 1.0 mm/h found in the inactive ankylosing spondylitis group.

For C-reactive protein levels, all three patient groups, active ankylosing spondylitis ($p < 0.001$, $t = 7.60$), inactive ankylosing spondylitis ($p < 0.05$, $t = 2.23$) and rheumatoid arthritis ($p < 0.001$, $t = 5.85$), had significantly higher levels than the one of 1.6 ± 0.6 μg/ml measured in the controls.

Furthermore, the inactive ankylosing spondylitis group had significantly lower C-reactive protein level compared to the active ankylosing spondylitis group ($p < 0.001$, $t = 5.87$) and the rheumatoid arthritis group ($p < 0.001$, $t = 3.23$).

The mean ($\pm$ standard error) serum IgG in active ankylosing spondylitis was 20.60 ± 0.15 g/l and this was significantly higher than the level of 14.04 ± 0.82 g/l found in inactive ankylosing spondylitis ($p < 0.001$, $t = 3.93$), the level of 15.20 ± 0.94 g/l found in the rheumatoid arthritis group ($p < 0.005$, $t = 3.15$) and the level of 12.44 ± 0.44 g/l found in the controls ($p < 0.001$, $t = 6.28$).

The mean ($\pm$ standard error) serum IgA of the active ankylosing spondylitis was 4.74 ± 0.24 g/l and this was significantly higher than the level of 2.55 ± 0.21 g/l found in the rheumatoid arthritis group ($p < 0.001$, $t = 6.82$) or the level of 1.96 ± 0.15 g/l found in the control group ($p < 0.001$, $t = 10.35$).

The mean ($\pm$ standard error) serum IgA of the rheumatoid arthritis group was 2.55 ± 0.21 g/l and this was significantly higher than the level of 1.74 ± 0.08 g/l found in the inactive ankylosing spondylitis group ($p < 0.001$, $t = 3.53$) or the level of 1.96 ± 0.15 g/l found in the control group ($p < 0.025$, $t = 2.34$).

Coombs Agglutination Assay

Proteus mirabilis (B17) and *Klebsiella pneumoniae var oxytoca* (MX100) were obtained from the Department of Microbiology at Queen Elizabeth College. The cultures were maintained on nutrient agar slopes at room temperature.

Nutrient broth (Oxoid) 13 g/l of water was autoclaved at 121°C, 1.05 kg/cm^2 for 15 min. A starter culture was prepared in 25 ml of autoclaved nutrient broth in a 250-ml conical flask and inoculated from the agar slope, incubated at 37°C for 6 h and agitated at 250 rpm on an orbital shaker.

Shake-flask cultures were prepared by inoculating 200 ml of nutrient broth, in a 2-l conical flask with 10-ml culture from the starter broth, incubated at 37°C and shaken for 16 h at 250 rpm on an orbital shaker.

Overnight cultures were centrifuged at $2,500 \times g$ for 15 min, washed three times with phosphate-buffered saline and the pellet resuspended in 25-ml phosphate-buffered saline.

The concentration of the bacteria was adjusted to give an optical density of 1.64 in a Spectrophotometer 1800 at 540 nm, since this had been found to give optimum agglutination. It was equivalent to 1.57×10^{12} cells/ml for *Klebsiella* and 2.05×10^{11} cells/ml for *Proteus* microorganisms, when measured in a Coulter counter (Model 2B1).

The agglutination assay was carried out as follows: 100 µl volumes of bacterial suspension were added to 100 µl doubling dilutions of test serum in Dreyer's tubes. The mixtures were incubated at 37°C for 2 h, then 350-µl phosphate-buffered saline was added and the tubes were centrifuged for 20 min ($1,500 \times g$, Mistral 6 l) at 4°C.

The supernatant was decanted, the pellet resuspended in 350-µl fresh phosphate-buffered saline, and the washing repeated twice. After the final wash, the pellet was resuspended in 100 µl one-tenth dilution in phosphate-buffered saline of Coombs rabbit anti-human immunoglobulin reagent. The tubes were incubated at 37°C for 2 h, then at 4°C overnight and the agglutination end-point determined.

All test serum samples were coded and end-points read blind, in that the tester was unaware whether patient or control sera were being investigated.

Results of Coombs agglutination Assay

Three separate agglutination studies were carried out against whole *Proteus mirabilis* and *Klebsiella pneumoniae var oxytoca* microorganisms. There were approximately 40 serum samples in each run, all tests were carried out blind and all samples came from different individuals. Therefore, each

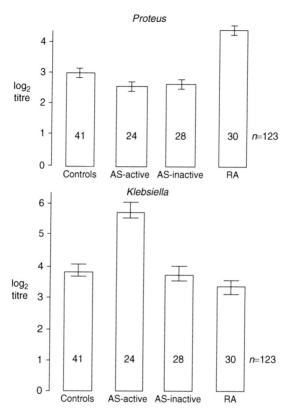

FIGURE 3.1 Antibody agglutination titres (mean ± standard error) from three pooled runs. Number of subjects in each group is indicated (Reprinted from Ebringer et al. (1985), with permission from Elsevier)

coded run was an independent investigation and the pooled results are shown (Fig. 3.1).

The mean (± standard error) *Proteus mirabilis* agglutination titre in the rheumatoid arthritis patients was 4.50 ± 0.18 $\log_2$ dilution units and this was significantly higher than the level of 3.08 ± 0.17 $\log_2$ dilution units found in the active ankylosing spondylitis group ($p<0.001, t=5.69$), the titre of 2.68 ± 0.16 $\log_2$

dilution units found in the inactive ankylosing spondylitis patients ($p < 0.001$, $t = 7.60$) or the level of $2.63 \pm 0.16 \log_2$ dilution units found in the healthy controls ($p < 0.001$, $t = 9.27$).

The mean ($\pm$ standard error) *Klebsiella pneumoniae* agglutination titre in the active ankylosing spondylitis patients was $5.80 \pm 0.20 \log_2$ dilution units and this was significantly higher than the level of $3.79 \pm 0.21 \log_2$ dilution units found in the inactive ankylosing spondylitis group ($p < 0.001$, $t = 6.26$), the titre of $3.67 \pm 0.24 \log_2$ dilution units in the rheumatoid arthritis patients ($p < 0.001$, $t = 7.22$) or the level of $3.85 \pm 0.15 \log_2$ dilution units in the healthy controls ($p < 0.001$, $t = 7.61$).

Clinical Implications and Discussion

The data presented here show that there are specific and significant antibody elevations against the urinary microbe *Proteus mirabilis* in rheumatoid arthritis patients attending the 'Gold Clinic' of the Middlesex Hospital in London when compared to active and inactive ankylosing spondylitis or healthy blood donors.

There are also specific and significant antibody elevations against the commensal bowel microbe *Klebsiella pneumoniae* in active ankylosing spondylitis patients from London when compared to rheumatoid arthritis patients or healthy blood donors.

The high level of *Proteus* antibodies in rheumatoid arthritis was not due to nonspecific effects of high immunoglobulin levels, since the patients with active ankylosing spondylitis had higher serum levels of IgG and IgA than the rheumatoid arthritis patients, yet their levels of *Proteus* antibodies were similar to those of inactive ankylosing spondylitis patients and healthy controls. To some extent, the two groups of patients with inflammatory arthritis acted as reciprocal controls to one another, in that rheumatoid arthritis patients had high levels of antibodies to *Proteus* but not against *Klebsiella* and active ankylosing spondylitis patients had high titres against *Klebsiella* but not against *Proteus*.

Inactive ankylosing spondylitis patients and healthy controls did not have high antibody titres against either microorganism.

It is relevant to note that inactive ankylosing spondylitis did not have elevated levels of anti-*Klebsiella* antibodies despite having bony changes and sacro-iliitis, features characteristic of the disease. The elevated antibody level to *Klebsiella* microbes is not associated with the phenotype of the disease but with the presence of inflammation.

These observations were published in 1985 and are the first report that active rheumatoid arthritis patients have elevated levels of antibodies to the microbe *Proteus mirabilis* which is known to cause upper urinary tract infections (Ebringer et al. 1985). Further studies are required to determine whether similar observations can be made in rheumatoid arthritis patients from other centres and different countries.

The rabbit antiserum produced against human HLA-DR4 lymphocytes indicated that some bacterial antigens especially from *Proteus* bacteria may carry epitopes resembling human HLA sequences. Clearly such a hypothesis requires also further investigations.

Proteus bacteria are widely distributed in the environment and can be isolated from soil, sputum and urinary cultures. Many different microbiological agents have been suggested in the past as possible exogenous factors in rheumatoid arthritis, such as diphtheroids, L-phase variants, mycoplasmas and a variety of viruses, but further examination failed to confirm the original observations (Marmion 1976). In a survey using direct agglutination of 30 microbiological agents in 22 newly diagnosed rheumatoid arthritis patients, some patients had responses against herpes virus hominis and *Proteus OXK* (Chandler et al. 1971).

One serious problem with these previous investigations is that an assumption is being made, that the external microbiological agent would target the joint and could be isolated from the synovial cavity. However, the possibility that an autologous agent, such as an antibody made by the rheumatoid arthritis patient being responsible for the joint inflammation, was not considered as a possibility. Yet this is exactly what happens in rheumatic fever: An infection by *Streptococcus pyogenes* located in the tonsils and upper respiratory tract evokes anti-bacterial antibodies which not only bind to the microbe wherever it is located but also to cross-reacting self-antigens found in the heart causing rheumatic fever and to the basal ganglia of the brain and giving rise to Sydenham's chorea.

During his first year residency, the author of this book witnessed a spectacular case of a 16-year-old female rheumatic fever patient with a pronounced heart murmur and severe chorea which prevented her from walking or going to the toilet and the attending senior physician made the confident claim that he would cure her in 1 week with the use of penicillin antibiotics. On the subsequent ward-round, 1 week later, the patient was running around filling the water bottles of the other elderly stroke female patients in the ward whose clinical status had not changed. If rheumatic fever could be caused by cross-reactive autologous antibodies evoked by an infection, why not other diseases?

Conclusions

Longitudinal studies are required in rheumatoid arthritis patients to assess whether antibiotic intervention will reduce the anti-*Proteus* antibody titre and modify the clinical outcome of the arthritic disease. The role of *Proteus* in rheumatoid arthritis patients merits further study.

References

Bennet PH, Wood PNH. Population studies of the rheumatic diseases. Amsterdam: Excerpta Medica; 1968. p. 456.

Chandler RW, Robinson H, Masi AT. Serological investigations for evidence of an infectious aetiology of rheumatoid arthritis. Ann Rheum Dis. 1971;30:274–8.

Cowling P, Ebringer R, Ebringer A. Association of inflammation with raised serum IgA in ankylosing spondylitis. Ann Rheum Dis. 1980;39:545–9.

Ebringer A, Ptaszynska T, Corbett M, Wilson C, Macafee Y, Avakian H, et al. Antibodies to *Proteus* in rheumatoid arthritis. Lancet. 1985;ii:305–7.

Marmion BP. A microbiologist's view of investigative rheumatology. In: Dumonde DC, editor. Infection and immunology in the rheumatic diseases. Oxford: Blackwell; 1976. p. 245–58.

Ropes MW, Bennett GA, Cobb S, Jacox R, Jessar RA. Revision of Diagnostic Criteria for Rheumatoid Arthritis. Bull Rheum Dis. 1958;9:175–6.

Chapter 4
Antibodies to *Proteus* in Irish Patients with Rheumatoid Arthritis

Contents

Ireland: An Introduction

Early in 1985, Mr. Alex Whelan, the chief technician from St. Vincent's Hospital in Dublin, in Ireland, came to the Department of Immunology at the Middlesex Hospital to study under Professor Ivan Roitt and to extend his knowledge of immunological techniques. He became familiar with the work of the Immunology Unit at King's College, but the patients with ankylosing spondylitis and rheumatoid arthritis

A. Ebringer, *Rheumatoid Arthritis and Proteus*,
DOI 10.1007/978-0-85729-950-5_4,
© Springer-Verlag London Limited 2012

patients were treated in the Department of Rheumatology at the Middlesex Hospital which was located a floor below the Department of Immunology.

When told that elevated levels of antibodies to *Proteus mirabilis* had been found in rheumatoid arthritis patients, Mr. Alex Whelan expressed the intention that he would propose an investigation of rheumatoid arthritis patients, under the care of Dr. Barry Bresnihan attending his hospital in Dublin for the presence or absence of antibodies to *Proteus mirabilis*.

Dublin: Location and History

Dublin is the capital and the largest city of the Republic of Ireland. It has a population of over one million and is located on the eastern side of the island. The name is derived from the Irish name 'Dubh Linn' which means 'black pool'. The town was established by the Norse Vikings in 841 AD. It was sacked by the Celtic king Brian Boru who defeated the Norse at the Battle of Clontarf in 1014. The Norman invasion of Ireland in 1170 opened up a relentless struggle over the centuries with the Anglo-Norman nobility which ended with the partition of Ireland in 1922 and the setting up of the Republic.

Patients and Controls

Patients with rheumatoid arthritis attending the Rheumatology Clinic of St. Vincents Hospital in Dublin were studied.

Patients with active rheumatoid arthritis, that is, those who were deemed to require sodium aurothiomalate or lymphoid irradiation, were investigated for the presence of antibodies to *Proteus mirabilis* and compared to patients with systemic lupus erythematosus or sarcoidosis, as well as healthy controls.

All 29 patients had definite or classical rheumatoid arthritis as defined by the American Rheumatism Association (Ropes et al. 1958). Ten rheumatoid arthritis patients were treated with gold sodium thiomalate, each patient receiving a cumulative dose of 1 g. Nineteen rheumatoid arthritis patients received lymphoid irradiation therapy (Hanly et al. 1986). These were randomly chosen to receive total doses of either 750 rad (9 patients) or 2,000 rad (10 patients) lymphoid irradiation. Radiotherapy was given on an outpatient basis four times weekly, using an 8 meV linear accelerator. Lymph nodes in the upper half of the body, which included the cervical, mediastinal and hilar lymph nodes, were encompassed in a mantle field and overall midline dose was given in 10 fractions. Without interruption, the lymph nodes in the lower half of the body, including the para-aortic, iliac and inguinal lymph nodes (inverted Y-field), received a similar midline dose in 10 fractions. The overall treatment was usually completed in 5–6 weeks. The spleen was not included in the radiation portal. Haemoglobin levels, white cell counts and platelet counts were monitored regularly during treatment.

In one premenopausal female patient, the pelvic lymph nodes were shielded to protect the ovaries.

Enzyme-Linked Immunosorbent Assay (ELISA)

The ELISA assays were performed either by the Biodot Microfiltration apparatus (Biorad) or the conventional 96 well microtitre plates (Nunc). Bacterial isolates of *Proteus mirabilis* were obtained from the Department of Microbiology, St. James Hospital in Dublin and grown on nutrient agar plates (Oxoid). The organisms were harvested and washed in 0.2 molar phosphate-buffered saline (PBS) pH 7.4 by centrifugation at 2,500 g for 20 min at 4°C.

Proteus sonicate was prepared by fixing the bacteria in 1% formaldehyde in PBS for 20 min. After washing twice in PBS, the organisms were sonicated and bacterial debris pelleted. The supernatant was removed and stored at 4°C. The *Proteus* sonicate was adjusted to give an optical density (OD) reading of 0.66 at 280 nm in 0.02 tris-buffered saline (BS) at pH 7.5 and 100 μl of this was incubated on nitrocellulose membrane for 10 min using the Biodot Microfiltration apparatus. After each incubation, the membrane was washed in 0.05% Tween-TBS (TTBS). The remaining binding sites were blocked by applying 100 μl of 3% bovine serum albumin (BSA) in TTBS to each well. The wells were washed a further five times and peroxidase-conjugated affinity purified goat anti-human IgG (Biorad) diluted 1/1,000 was then applied in 100 μl volumes for 30 min at room temperature. The nitrocellulose sheet was then removed from the apparatus, washed and incubated for 3 min in an acetate buffer 0.02 M, pH 5.1 containing 3-amino-9-ethylcarbazole (EAC) in 0.02% H_2O_2. The reaction was stopped by washing with distilled water, and the sheet was then allowed to dry overnight in the dark. Each lane was scanned using a transmittance/reflectometer scanning densitometer in the reflectance mode.

When microtitre plates were used, *Proteus* sonicate was adjusted to give an optical density (OD) of 1.6 at 280 nm while whole organisms were adjusted to a concentration of 6.4×10^6 organisms/ml in carbonate/bicarbonate buffer pH 9.6. Hundred microliter aliquots of either sonicate or whole *Proteus* was then added to the microtitre wells and incubated overnight at 4°C. Wells coated with sonicate were washed twice with PBS/Tween and blocked with 3% BSA in PBS for 1 h at room temperature, whereas the wells coated with whole *Proteus* were blocked with 1% gelatin for the same period after the initial two washes.

Serum samples were diluted 1/50 in PBS/Tween for the sonicate assay and 1/25 when using whole *Proteus* bacteria. Hundred microliter volumes of each dilution were added to each well for 30 min and incubated for 37°C. Following three washes, commercially available peroxidase-conjugated rabbit anti-human IgG (Dako) was diluted 1/500 in PBS/Tween and 100 μl volumes added. After 30 min incubation at 37°C, the plates were washed again in PBS/Tween. Hundred microliter of substrate *o*-phenylenediamine (OPD) was then added to each well and the reaction stopped after 15 min with the addition of 2.5 M H_2SO_4. The microtitre plates were read on a Dynatech spectrophotometer at wavelength 490 nm.

Results of the Assays

Results with Sonicated Proteus Antigen

When sonicated *Proteus* organisms were used as the antigen to detect antibodies in rheumatoid arthritis patients or control subjects, prior to treatment using the dot or microtitre ELISA assays, no significant difference was found between the two groups.

However, in rheumatoid arthritis patients after gold treatment, a fall in anti-*Proteus* antibodies was observed using both of these assay systems. This reduction reached significance with the microtitre ELISA technique ($p < 0.02$). No fall in antibody levels was seen in patients after the lymphoid irradiation.

Results with Whole Proteus Bacteria

However, when whole *Proteus* bacteria was used as a target, there was a significant difference in antibody levels ($p < 0.01$) between controls and rheumatoid arthritis patients before treatment.

Again, there was a significant fall in these antibody levels after gold therapy ($p < 0.01$), but there was no fall observed after lymphoid irradiation.

The levels of antibodies to *Proteus* in rheumatoid arthritis patients were significantly elevated ($p < 0.001$) when compared to healthy blood donors as well as when compared to the three disease groups: coeliac disease, sarcoidosis, systemic lupus erythematosus patients (Fig. 4.1).

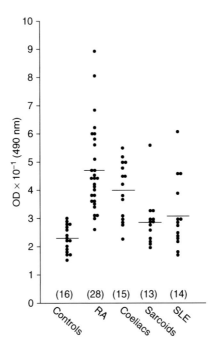

FIGURE 4.1 IgG anti-*Proteus mirabilis* antibody levels to whole *Proteus* bacteria as antigen using microtitre ELISA plates. The groups studied include normal controls ($n = 16$); active rheumatoid arthritis (28); coeliac disease ($n = 15$); sarcoidosis ($n = 13$) and systemic lupus erythematosus ($n = 14$) patients. Each *dot* represents either a control subject or a patient (Reprinted from Rogers et al. 1988, with permission from Oxford University Press)

Of the three disease control groups, only patients with coeliac disease had significantly elevated levels of antibodies against *Proteus* when compared to healthy blood donors ($p < 0.01$) but the level observed was nevertheless lower than that seen in patients with rheumatoid arthritis.

Clinical Implications and Discussion

Patients with active rheumatoid arthritis patients showed significant elevations in IgG antibody against whole *Proteus* bacteria when compared to patients with coeliac disease, sarcoidosis and systemic lupus as well as to healthy blood donors.

There was also a rise in the anti-*Proteus* antibody titre in coeliac disease when compared to healthy controls and this may reflect some gut mucosal damage. The presence of increased α-gliadin antibodies in rheumatoid arthritis patients has been reported (O'Farrell et al. 1986).

The results with sonicated *Proteus* antigen were equivocal which suggests that the assay conditions may have not been optimized for this study.

The results in the rheumatoid arthritis pre- and post-irradiation lymphoid irradiation showed no correlation between clinical improvement and *Proteus* antibody levels.

However, in the gold treated group, there was a reduction in *Proteus* antibody levels following drug therapy. The Dublin group had previously reported that IgG, IgM and IgM RF levels fall following gold therapy (Hassan et al. 1984; Hanly et al. 1985). Thus, the reduced anti-*Proteus* antibody level may be a result of the general reduction in immunoglobulins.

The possibility of 'rheumatoid factor' amplifying the results by binding to specific *Proteus* antibodies in the assay systems was investigated.Rheumatoid arthritis sera were absorbed to remove 'rheumatoid factor' using latex particles coated with human IgG. The results of these studies did not reveal any interference in the assay systems.

In conclusion, increased anti-*Proteus* antibody levels were found in Irish patients with rheumatoid arthritis, to a lesser extent in patients with coeliac disease when compared to patients with sarcoidosis or systemic lupus erythematosus or healthy blood donors. These results confirm the results obtained by the London group.

These results were presented by Mr. Alex Whelan at the 'Second International Symposium' held at the Middlesex Hospital on 14–15 April 1987 (Ebringer and Shipley 1988).

During the discussion at this meeting, Mr. Alex Whelan expressed the following comment:

> The whole story about *Proteus* has potential interest only if you find crossreactivity to other agents. There appears to be an indication for a possible aetiological agent coming from the gut. If you then ask the question, which has probably been asked many times over the last two centuries, if there is an agent in rheumatoid arthritis, is it very rare or very common?
>
> If it is very rare, we would possibly have found it. If it is very common, it is because we all have it. Then if you ask the question what does genetic susceptibility mean, unless someone gives me a better answer, I think "molecular mimicry" stands out OK (Rogers et al. 1988).

References

Ebringer A, Shipley M, editors. Pathogenesis of ankylosing spondylitis and rheumatoid arthritis. Br J Rheum. 1988;27(Suppl. II):1–178.

Hanly J, Hassan J, Whelan A, Feighery C, Bresnihan B. The effect of gold therapy on rheumatoid factor synthesis by synovial membrane. Br J Rheumatol. 1985;24:103.

Hanly JG, Hassan J, Moriarty M, Barry C, Molony J, Casey E, et al. Lymphoid irradiation in intractable rheumatoid arthritis. A double-blind randomized study comparing 750-rad treatment with 2,000 rad treatment. Arthritis Rheum. 1986;29:16–25.

Hassan J, Hanly J, Whelan A, Feighery C, Bresnihan B. In-vitro production of immunoglobulins in patients with active rheumatoid arthritis and changes with gold therapy. Irish J Med Sci. 1984; 153:256.

O'Farrell C, Price R, Fernandes L. Immune sensitization to dietary antigens associated with IgA rheumatoid factor in rheumatoid arthritis. Br J Rheumatol. 1986;Abstract (Suppl. 2), Abs. 89.

Rogers P, Hassan J, Bresnihan B, Feighery C, Whelan A. Antibodies to *Proteus* in rheumatoid arthritis. Br J Rheumatol. 1988;27(Suppl II): 90–4.

Ropes MW, Bennett GA, Cobb S, Jacox R, Jessar R. 1958 revision of diagnostic criteria for rheumatoid arthritis. Bull Rheum Dis. 1958;9:175–6.

Chapter 5
Antibodies to *Proteus* in Rheumatoid Arthritis Patients from Bermuda and from Hertfordshire in England

Contents

A. Ebringer, *Rheumatoid Arthritis and Proteus*,
DOI 10.1007/978-0-85729-950-5_5,
© Springer-Verlag London Limited 2012

Bermuda and Hertfordshire: Introduction

In 1992, during one of his visits back to Bermuda, Dr. Clyde Wilson met the physician Dr. Henry Subair who expressed an interest in the work of the 'Immunology Unit' at King's College in London. He mentioned that he had patients suffering from rheumatoid arthritis especially women and would be willing to participate in a study to investigate whether his Bermudian patients had similar antibodies to the ones described in English patients with rheumatoid arthritis from London.

It was decided to compare Bermudian rheumatoid arthritis patients with a group of English rheumatoid arthritis patients attending the Lister Hospital in Stevenage under the medical care of Dr. Allan Binder. The Lister Hospital has 600–700 beds and is located in Hertfordshire which is a county of south-east England, lying just north of Greater London. Most of the rheumatoid arthritis patients in the Lister hospital came from northern Hertfordshire, namely, Stevenage, Hitchin and Letchworth.

Both groups of rheumatoid arthritis patients were studied under blind conditions in that the person doing the antibody assays did not know which samples came from Bermuda or Hertfordshire and which came from patients or healthy donors.

The antibody studies were carried out by two different techniques ELISA and immunofluorescence.

Bermuda: Location and History

Bermuda is a small but prosperous island located some 1,000 miles north-east from Miami in the Atlantic. It was discovered in 1505 by the Spanish explorer Juan de Bermudez who gave the island its name. The island was settled by England in 1609, making it the oldest British overseas territory. It has a mild subtropical climate which accounts for its attraction to visitors. It is a centre of finance and tourism which provides its multi-ethnic population of over 60,000 with a high standard of living.

It has one of the highest GDP (Gross Domestic Product) per capita in the world. Its old capital of St.George's was established in 1612 and is one of the oldest continuously inhabited English-speaking town in the Americas. The current capital is Hamilton where Dr. Henry Subair has his medical practice in the King Edward VII Memorial Hospital.

Bermuda has at its head a Governor appointed by the Crown, but since 1960, it is essentially a self-governing territory and forms part of the 'Caribbean Community'.

Patients and Controls

All the rheumatoid arthritis sera from both Bermuda and Hertfordshire were selected on the basis of clinical assessment of disease activity by the attending physicians and an elevated erythrocyte sedimentation rate (ESR) greater than 15 mm/h and a C-reactive protein level (CRP) greater than 10 mg/l.

It had previously been reported that patients with rheumatoid arthritis in the active phase of the disease, as measured by C-reactive protein levels, have higher levels of anti-*Proteus* antibodies compared to patients with inactive rheumatoid arthritis (Deighton et al. 1992).

Sera from Hamilton, Bermuda

Sera were obtained from 34 patients with active rheumatoid arthritis (5 male/29 female) attending the King Edward VII Memorial Hospital in Hamilton, Bermuda with a mean age of 56.9 years (range = 32–79 years) having a mean erythrocyte sedimentation rate (± standard error) of 40.5 ± 5.1 mm/h. The female/male ratio in the rheumatoid arthritis patients from Bermuda was 5.8. Samples were also obtained from 33 healthy controls (5 male/28 female) having a mean age of

57.1 years (range: 32–79 years). Erythrocyte sedimentation rates were not measured in the controls.

Sera from Stevenage, Hertfordshire

Sera were also collected from 34 patients with active rheumatoid arthritis (8 male/26 female) attending the Rheumatology Department of the Lister Hospital in Stevenage, Hertfordshire with a mean age of 59.0 years (range = 21–83 years) having a mean erythrocyte sedimentation rate (± standard error) of 49.6 ± 4.8 mm/h. The female/male ratio in the rheumatoid arthritis patients from Hertfordshire was 3.3. Erythrocyte sedimentation rates were not measured in the controls.

Preparation of the Bacteria for the ELISA Study

Bacterial isolates of *Proteus mirabilis* and *Escherichia coli* were obtained from the Department of Microbiology at King's College and prepared as previously published.

The cultures were grown aerobically in 250-ml conical flasks on an orbital shaker for 16–18 h in nutrient broth (Oxoid 13 g/l). Inoculation was performed by the addition of one loopful of bacteria from a nutrient agar plate. The cells were harvested by centrifugation at 4°C at 6,000 rpm for 20 min (MSE 18.6×250 ml rotor).

Bacterial isolates of three components of normal bowel flora were also obtained. A faecal sample was collected from a healthy adult and processed with careful attention to anaerobic technique. Isolates were identified by gram reaction, morphology and end product analysis by gas liquid chromatography (Borriello et al. 1978). Selected biochemical tests were also carried out using the rapid identification system (Rapid ID-32A, API Biomérieux).

The three normal bow el flora isolates were *Eubacterium* sp (Strain NF-iii), *Peptostreptococcus* sp (NF-ii-a) and *Bacteroides fragilis* (NF-vii).

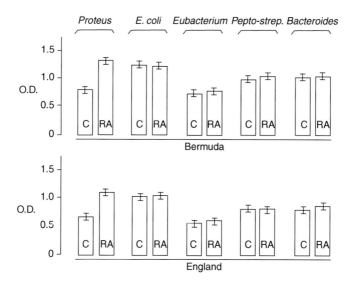

FIGURE 5.1 Antibody titres (mean±standard error) measured by ELISA to the indicated organisms in 34 Bermudian and 34 English patients with rheumatoid arthritis and 33 Bermudian and 30 English controls (*OD* optical density) (Reprinted from Subair et al. (1995), with kind permission from The Journal of Rheumatology)

ELISA Studies with Five Bacteria: *Proteus mirabilis*, *Escherichia coli* and Three Normal Bowel Flora Isolates *Eubacterium*, *Peptostreptococcus* and *Bacteroides*

ELISA investigations were carried under code using the method of Khalafpour (Khalafpour et al. 1988).

The Bermudian rheumatoid arthritis patients with active disease had an elevated level mean (± standard error) of IgG *Proteus* antibodies of 1.31 ± 0.04 OD units when compared to the level in Bermudian control subjects of 0.98 ± 0.04 OD units and this difference was highly significant ($t = 6.07$, $p < 0.001$) (Fig. 5.1).

TABLE 5.1 Comparison of anti-*Proteus mirabilis* antibody titers (optical density or OD units) (Mean±standard error) in male and female rheumatoid arthritis (RA) patients and controls from Bermuda

Sex	Number	Status	Antibody level	Statistical significance
Male	5	RA	1.14 ± 0.08	$P < 0.001$
	5	Controls	0.79 ± 0.09	
Female	29	RA	1.34 ± 0.04	$P < 0.001$
	28	Controls	1.01 ± 0.04	

The Hertfordshire rheumatoid arthritis patients with active disease also had an elevated level mean (± standard error) of IgG *Proteus* antibodies of 1.12 ± 0.03 OD units when compared to the level in English control subjects of 0.67 ± 0.03 OD units and this difference was again highly significant ($t = 9.77, p < 0.001$) (Fig. 5.1).

However, there was no significant elevation in IgG antibody titres in Bermudian or English patients with rheumatoid against *Escherichia coli* or total Ig against the three normal flora isolates, *Eubacterium* sp., *Peptostreptococcus* sp. and *Bacteroides fragilis*.

There was also a significant elevation in *Proteus* antibody titres in Bermudian men and women with rheumatoid arthritis when compared respectively to healthy Bermudian men and women (Table 5.1).

There was also a significant elevation of *Proteus* antibody titres in English men and women from Hertfordshire suffering from rheumatoid arthritis when compared to healthy English men and women respectively (Table 5.2).

There was no significant difference between men and women with rheumatoid arthritis either from Bermuda or Hertfordshire compared to their respective controls, when tested against the four other bacteria, namely *Escherichia coli* and the three normal bowel flora isolates *Eubacterium*, *Peptostreptococcus* and *Bacteroides fragilis*.

TABLE 5.2 Comparison of anti-*Proteus mirabilis* antibody titers (optical density or OD units) (Mean ± standard error) in male and female rheumatoid arthritis (RA) patients and controls from England

Sex	Number	Status	Antibody level	Statistical significance
Male	8	RA	1.09 ± 0.03	P < 0.001
	15	Controls	0.65 ± 0.06	
Female	29	RA	1.13 ± 0.04	P < 0.001
	28	Controls	0.71 ± 0.04	

Indirect Immunofluorescence Studies with *Proteus* in Both Bermudian and Hertfordshire Rheumatoid Arthritis Patients

Indirect immunofluorescence studies were carried out on the same 34 Bermudian patients with rheumatoid arthritis and controls but compared to a new batch of 30 rheumatoid arthritis from Hertfordshire.

The reason for using new sera in the English test and controls between ELISA and indirect immunofluorescence was due to inadequate volumes of sera available for both assays.

Indirect immunofluorescence was only used with *Proteus mirabilis* which was cultured as described previously. However, before dilution, a 1-ml aliquot of the stock bacterial solution was mixed with 1 ml of glutaraldehyde (0.25% v/v Sigma) in PBS to fix the bacteria.

The resulting suspension was then left for 10 min, and after this time, the dilution process was carried as before. Aliquots of 10 μl of the diluted bacterial suspension were added to each of the eight wells on the glass slide (ICN Flow Labs). The slides were then incubated at 30°C for 20 min to allow the bacteria to adhere to the glass slide. A 10-μl aliquot of test or control serum serially diluted from 1:10 through to 1:1,280 with *Proteus mirabilis* as the antigen in PBS (0.15 M, pH 7.4) was added to each well and incubated in a damp box for 1 h. Each serum sample was tested in duplicate. The slides were then washed in a bath of PBS, continually stirred with a magnetic flea for 30 min at room temperature. After washing, the slides were carefully dried all around the wells using a cotton bud. Then 15 µl of rabbit anti-human IgG antibody conjugated to fluorescein isothiocyanate (FITC) (Dako Ltd), diluted 1:20 in PBS, was added to each test area. The slides were then incubated for a further 30 min at room temperature in a damp box followed by washing for 1 h, dried, 10 µl of mounting fluid (Sigma) was added to each test area, a cover slip applied and fixed using clear nail varnish around the edges.

Viewing of the test area was carried out using an immunofluorescence microscope (Leitz Dialux 20) with a 100× Leitz lens under water immersion. Each sample was scored between 0 and 8 $\log_2$ dilution units depending on the end point of fluorescence. No fluorescence at a dilution of 1: 10 scored a value of zero, fluorescence at 1: 10 scored 1, fluorescence at 1: 20 scored 2 and so on, up to a value up to a value of 1: 1,280 which scored 8. The results were expressed as anti-*Proteus* antibody titre ± standard error (IIFA units).

All runs were carried out under code in that the microscopist was not aware of the status of the sera under examination.

The indirect immunofluorescence studies confirmed the results obtained by the ELISA technique in that both the Bermudian and Herfordshire rheumatoid arthritis patients had elevated levels of antibodies to *Proteus mirabilis* when compared to their respective controls.

The 34 Bermudian rheumatoid arthritis patients with active disease had an elevated level mean (± standard error) of IgG antibodies to *Proteus mirabilis* of 6.06 ± 0.28 IIFA units when compared to the level in 33 in Bermudian control subjects of 2.86 ± 0.21 and this difference was highly significant ($t = 9.26, p < 0.001$) (Fig. 5.2).

The 31 rheumatoid arthritis patients with active disease from Hertfordshire had an elevated level mean (± standard

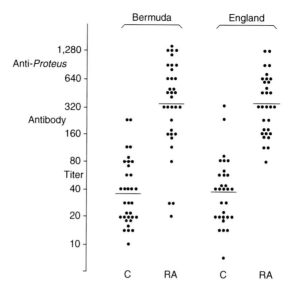

FIGURE 5.2 IgG antibody titres to *Proteus mirabilis* in 34 Bermudian and 31 English patients with rheumatoid arthritis and 33 Bermudian and 30 English controls measured by indirect immunofluorescence assay. (Bar = mean). Each *dot* represents the serum of either a rheumatoid arthritis patient or a blood donor subject (Reprinted from Subair et al. (1995), with kind permission from The Journal of Rheumatology)

error) of IgG antibodies to *Proteus mirabilis* of 6.06 ± 0.20 when compared to the level in 30 blood donor subjects of 2.88 ± 0.22 and again this difference was highly significant ($t = 10.94, p < 0.001$) (Fig. 5.2).

Clinical Implications

The results, by using two different techniques, show that both Bermudian and English rheumatoid arthritis patients from northern Hertfordshire have specific antibody elevations against *Proteus mirabilis.*

Furthermore, the ELISA studies show that this elevation is not present against *Escherichia coli* or three normal bowel bacteria. This confirms our previous report and the findings of the Newcastle group in England (Deighton et al. 1992) regarding the specificity of the anti-*Proteus* antibody elevation in rheumatoid arthritis patients.

The demonstration of a significant IgG antibody to *Proteus mirabilis* but not to the four other bacteria clearly eliminates the suggestion that rheumatoid arthritis patients have a 'leaky gut'. The 'leaky gut' hypothesis proposes that prolonged use of non-steroidal anti-inflammatory drugs (NSAIDS) causes increased gut permeability to bowel bacteria or antigens and this might explain the elevation in anti-*Proteus* antibodies (Bjarnason et al. 1984).

If NSAID-induced gut ulceration was responsible for the increased level of anti-*Proteus* antibodies found in rheumatoid arthritis patients, then an antibody elevation to common bowel bacteria such as *Escherichia coli* or the three normal bowel isolates would also have been detected. The number of microorganisms per gram of faeces is of the order of 10^{12} for anaerobic bacteria, 10^8 for *Escherichia coli* but only 10^7 microbes per gram of faeces for *Proteus mirabilis* (Hentges 1983; Drasar and Barrow 1985).

Clearly, the lack of any immune response to *Escherichia coli* and the three normal bowel bacteria suggests that NSAID-induced increased gut permeability is not the explanation for the elevation of anti-*Proteus* antibodies found in rheumatoid arthritis patients.

Proteus mirabilis can be isolated from about 10% of patients with a urinary tract infection (Guenzel 1986). Since women suffer from 'urinary tract infections' more frequently than men, this could explain the higher prevalence of rheumatoid arthritis in the female population throughout the world. Indeed it has been reported that rheumatoid arthritis patients suffer from an increased incidence of 'urinary tract infections' (Tishler et al. 1992).

The results of the Bermudian and Hertfordshire study have been published, and a copy of the paper has been deposited in the Historical Archives of Bermuda (Subair et al. 1995).

The data presented here show that there are specific and significant antibody elevations against *Proteus mirabilis* in rheumatoid arthritis patients in both the Western (Bermuda) and Eastern Hemispheres (Northern Hertfordshire, England).

References

Bjarnason I, Williams P, So A, Zanelli GD, Levi AJ, Gumpel JM, et al. Intestinal permeability and inflammation in rheumatoid arthritis: effects of non-steroidal anti-inflammatory drugs. Lancet. 1984;2:1171–3.

Borriello SP, Hudson MJ, Hill MJ. Investigation of the gastrointestinal bacterial flora. Clin Gastroenterol. 1978;7:329–49.

Deighton CM, Gray J, Bint AJ, Walker DJ. Specificity of the *Proteus* antibody response in rheumatoid arthritis. Ann Rheum Dis. 1992;51:1206–7.

Drasar BS, Barrow PA. Intestinal microbiology. 3rd ed. Wokingham: Van Nostrand Reinhold; 1985.

Guenzel MN. *Escherichia*, *Klebsiella*, *Enterobacter*, *Serratia*, *Citrobacter* and *Proteus*. In: Baron S, editor. Medical microbiology. 2nd ed. Menlo Park: Addison Wesley; 1986. p. 495–506.

Hentges DJ. Human intestinal microflora in health and disease. Chapter 1. New York: Academic; 1983.

Khalafpour S, Ebringer A, Abuljadayel I, Corbett M. Antibodies to *Klebsiella* and *Proteus* microorganisms in ankylosing spondylitis and rheumatoid arthritis patients measured by ELISA. Br J Rheumatol. 1988;27 Suppl 2:86–9.

Subair H, Tiwana H, Fielder M, Binder A, Cunningham P, Ebringer A, et al. Elevation in anti-*Proteus* antibodies in patients with rheumatoid arthritis from Bermuda and England. J Rheumatol. 1995;22:1825–8.

Tishler M, Caspi D, Aimog Y, Segal R, Yaron M. Increased incidence of urinary tract infection in patients with rheumatoid arthritis and secondary Sjögren's syndrome. Ann Rheum Dis. 1992;51:604–6.

Chapter 6
Antibodies to *Proteus* in Rheumatoid Arthritis Patients from Brest and Toulouse in France

Contents

A. Ebringer, *Rheumatoid Arthritis and Proteus*,
DOI 10.1007/978-0-85729-950-5_6,
© Springer-Verlag London Limited 2012

Brest and Toulouse: Introduction

In the early 1990s, Professor Pierre Youinou from the University of Brest in France carried out collaborative studies on lymphocytes with Professor Ivan Roitt, in the Department of Immunology at the Middlesex Hospital in London. He came to know the work being carried out by the King's College Immunology group on *Proteus* antibodies in English patients and asked whether this was a general observation which applied to rheumatoid arthritis patients in different countries. He was interested in the question if similar observations could be made on French patients suffering from rheumatoid arthritis. He said that he could obtain sera from rheumatoid arthritis patients in Brest and also from a colleague Dr. A. Cantagrel in Toulouse, in south-western France and would provide control sera from the Blood Bank in Brest. However, he insisted that he would code the sera himself in France before they were dispatched to the UK. The studies would be carried out in London, results then sent back to France, decoded and the appropriate calculations carried out.

It was decided to compare rheumatoid arthritis patients from Brest and Toulouse to a set of control sera supplied by the Blood Bank in Brest.

The antibody studies were carried out by two different techniques, ELISA and immunofluorescence, on the Brest rheumatoid arthritis patients. The sera from patients with rheumatoid arthritis from Toulouse were tested only by immunofluorescence.

Brest: Location and History

Brest is located at the western tip of France and has a wide bay which makes it a natural harbour. The town has a population of 150,000 but provides services to about 1 million inhabitants of western Brittany. The city was almost completely destroyed during the Second World War because it was an important submarine base but has been largely rebuilt.

Brittany was an independent Duchy in the Middle Ages but was brought to the French crown as a dowry by the marriage of Anne de Bretagne to the French King.

Some 200,000 inhabitants of Brittany speak Breton, a Celtic language related to Cornish and Welsh, and there are strong cultural links with Wales, Galicia and Ireland.

Toulouse: Location and History

Toulouse is situated in south-western France on the banks of the Garonne river. It has been inhabited for almost 3,000 years, and during Roman times, it was known as Tolosa. It has a population of over 1 million. Its university is one of the oldest in Europe having been founded in 1229. During the early Middle Ages, it was the centre of a Visigothic empire stretching from southern Spain to northern France. More recently, it was the capital of the Languedoc region.

Hopital de Rangueil is situated in a university campus in Toulouse where Dr. A. Cantagrel was involved in rheumatological services. He provided the sera from 15 active rheumatoid arthritis patients to be studied by immunofluorescence for the presence of anti-*Proteus* antibodies.

Patients and Controls

All the rheumatoid arthritis sera from both Brest and Toulouse were selected on the basis of clinical assessment of disease activity by the attending physicians and an elevated erythrocyte sedimentation rate (ESR) greater than 15 mm/h.

Sera from Brest

Sera from 50 tissue-typed, active rheumatoid arthritis patients and 49 healthy controls were obtained from the Laboratoire d'Immunologie et de Rhumatologie, Centre Hospitalier

Régional et Universitaire (CHRU) from Brest in France. Patients were tissue typed by the micro-cyto-toxicity assay of Terasaki using standard reagents (France-Transplant). The characteristics of the Brest patients and controls were as follows. The mean age of the rheumatoid arthritis group was 60 years (range 14–84). In the rheumatoid arthritis patients, the mean erythrocyte sedimentation rate (± standard error) was 70.0 ± 3.0 mm/h. The female/male ratio in the rheumatoid arthritis patients from Brest was 2.3. The female/male ratio in the healthy controls was 2.8. Erythrocyte sedimentation rates were not measured in the controls. The percentage of rheumatoid arthritis–associated tissue types (DRB1*0101 (DR1) and DR4 combined) was 60%. Additionally, 8% of the rheumatoid arthritis patients carried HLA-B27. Control subjects were not tissue typed.

Sera from Toulouse

Sera were also collected from 15 patients with active rheumatoid arthritis attending the Rheumatology Department of the Rangueil Hospital in Toulouse. The rheumatoid arthritis patients from Toulouse were not tissue typed and the sera were used only for immunofluorescence studies.

ELISA Studies with Three Bacteria: *Proteus mirabilis*, *Escherichia coli* and *Salmonella typhimurium*

The ELISA studies, involving three different bacteria, *Proteus mirabilis*, *Escherichia coli* and *Salmonella typhimurium*, were carried out only on the rheumatoid arthritis sera from Brest, as previously described (Fielder et al. 1995).

The active rheumatoid arthritis patients from Brest had an elevated level mean (± standard error) of IgG *Proteus* antibodies of 1.156 ± 0.068 OD units when compared to the level in control subjects of 0.730 ± 0.160 OD units and this difference was statistically significant ($t = 4.24, p < 0.001$) (Fig. 6.1).

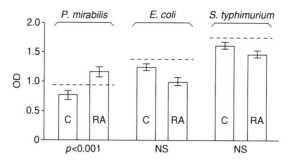

FIGURE 6.1 Antibody titres (mean ± standard error) for IgG in 49 controls (C) and 50 active rheumatoid arthritis patients (RA) from Brest when tested by ELISA, under code, against *Proteus mirabilis*, *Escherichia coli* and *Salmonella typhimurium*. (*Dotted line* indicates 95% confidence limits for mean of controls – one-tailed test; OD optical density) (Reprinted from Fielder et al. (1995), with permission from Springer Science + Business Media)

However, there was no significant elevation in IgG antibody titres in rheumatoid arthritis patients from Brest against *Escherichia coli* or *Salmonella typhimurium*.

Serum C-reactive protein level was measured in the Brest patients and controls by the radial immunodiffusion method of Mancini (Mancini et al. 1965).

The mean (± standard error) C-reactive protein level in the rheumatoid arthritis patients was 57.6 ± 5.0 mg/l, whilst in the control subjects, it was 18.7 ± 5.7 mg/l, and this difference was statistically significant ($t = 5.12$, $p < 0.001$).

Indirect Immunofluorescence Studies with *Proteus* in Rheumatoid Arthritis Patients from Brest and Toulouse

Serum anti-*Proteus* antibodies in 50 rheumatoid arthritis patients from Brest and 15 rheumatoid arthritis patients from Toulouse were measured by indirect immunofluorescence as previously described. The results were scored as follows: A score of zero was given for no fluorescence at a serum dilution of 1/10, whilst fluorescence at 1/10 scored 1, fluorescence at 1/20 scored 2, fluorescence at 1/40 scored 3, fluorescence at 1/80 scored 4 and so on up to a value of 1/1280 which scored 8. The results were described as $\log_2$ dilution units. The studies were again carried out under code in that the person doing the assay did not know which sera came from rheumatoid arthritis patients and which came from control subjects.

The mean ($\pm$ standard error) anti-*Proteus* antibody titre in the rheumatoid arthritis patients from Brest was 6.51 ± 0.16 whilst the mean ($\pm$ standard error) in the blood donors was 3.70 ± 0.16 and this difference was statistically significant ($t = 8.96$, $p < 0.001$) (Fig. 6.2).

The mean ($\pm$ standard error) anti-*Proteus* antibody titre in the rheumatoid arthritis patients from Toulouse was 6.30 ± 0.34 and this difference was again statistically significant when compared to the blood donors from Brest ($t = 4.96$, $p < 0.001$) (Fig. 6.2).

These results suggest that French rheumatoid arthritis patients, at least from Brest and Toulouse, also have specific elevations in antibody levels against *Proteus* microbes (Fielder et al. 1994).

The indirect immunofluorescence studies confirmed the results obtained by the ELISA technique in that French rheumatoid arthritis patients have elevated levels of antibodies to *Proteus* when compared to their respective national blood donor controls (Fielder et al. 1995).

Clinical Implications

The results by using two different techniques show that rheumatoid arthritis patients from Brest have specific antibody elevations against the urinary microbe *Proteus mirabilis* but not against *Escherichia coli* and *Salmonella typhimurium*. These results together with the immunofluorescence data from Toulouse confirm the previous studies from London, Dublin in Ireland,

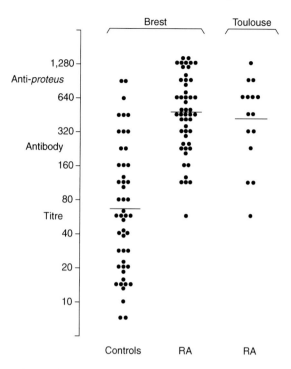

FIGURE 6.2 Antibody titres (bar = mean) for IgG in 49 controls and 50 active rheumatoid arthritis patients from Brest and 15 rheumatoid arthritis patients from Toulouse when tested by indirect immunofluorescence assay against *Proteus mirabilis*. Each *dot* represents the serum of either a rheumatoid arthritis patient or a blood donor subject (Reprinted from Fielder et al. (1995), with permission from Springer Science + Business Media)

Newcastle in England and Bermuda as well as northern Hertfordshire in that active rheumatoid arthritis patients have antibodies against a specific urinary pathogen *Proteus mirabilis*.

Furthermore, the ELISA studies show that this elevation is not present against *Escherichia coli*, a microbe involved frequently in causing cystitis especially in women.

References

Fielder M, Youinou P, Cantagrel A, Wilson C, Ebringer A. Elevation of anti-*Proteus* antibody titres in rheumatoid arthritis patients from Brest and Toulouse measured by immunofluorescence: a coded study. Clin Exp Rheumatol. 1994;12(Suppl II):S104, Abst C125.

Fielder M, Tiwana H, Youinou P, Le Goff P, Deonarain R, Wilson C, et al. The specificity of the of anti-*Proteus* antibody response in tissue typed rheumatoid arthritis patients from Brest. Rheumatol Int. 1995;15:79–82.

Mancini G, Carbonara HO, Heremans JF. Immunological quantification of antigens by single radial immunodiffusion. Immunochemistry. 1965;2:235–53.

Chapter 7
Dutch Patients with Rheumatoid Arthritis Have Antibodies to *Proteus*

Contents

The Netherlands Connection: An Introduction

In the early 1980s, the Immunology Unit of King's College had shown that there were elevated levels of antibodies to the Gram-negative bowel microbe *Klebsiella* in patients suffering from ankylosing spondylitis.

A. Ebringer, *Rheumatoid Arthritis and Proteus*,
DOI 10.1007/978-0-85729-950-5_7,
© Springer-Verlag London Limited 2012

In 1992, I was attending a Rheumatology Congress in Barcelona when the late Professor Bert Feltkamp from Amsterdam approached me and said: 'Alan, we have done 3 studies in the Netherlands and we cannot find antibodies in our Dutch ankylosing spondylitis patients as you do in London. It must be the London water'. Clearly, here was a challenge as I knew there was nothing wrong with the London water.

I said: 'Bert, you code the Dutch ankylosing spondylitis and uveitis patients in Amsterdam and send them to us in London. We will send you the results back to Amsterdam and you can decode them'.

'For good measure, send us also sera from active, rheumatoid arthritis patients who have an erythrocyte sedimentation rate greater than 30 mm/h (ESR > 30 mm/h) at the time the blood sample is taken, as we have also found the probable cause of this disease'.

'It is caused by a urinary tract infection by *Proteus* bacteria'. The sera were sent and the studies were carried out, using an immunofluorescence assay. For ankylosing spondylitis, we used an IgA anti-*Klebsiella* assay, whilst for rheumatoid arthritis, we used an IgG anti-*Proteus* assay.

Amsterdam: Location and History

Amsterdam is the capital and largest city of the Netherlands with a population of about two million. The city is in the province of North Holland, but the Ophthalmic Research Institute collects patients from the whole of the Netherlands.

Its name is derived from Amstellerdam, the city on the dam of the river Amstel. It started as a fishing village, but in 1306 was granted city rights. It is not as old as other Dutch cities such as Rotterdam, Utrecht and Nijmegen. However, it flourished in the Middle Ages, because it traded with the Hanseatic League.

In the sixteenth century, the Dutch rebelled against Philip II of Spain which led to the 'Eighty Years War' at the end of which Netherlands gained its independence.

The seventeenth century is considered Amsterdam's 'Golden Age' when it traded all over the world.

The Amsterdam merchants founded the Dutch East India Company and opened the first stock exchange in the world.

During the Second World War, the Dutch people suffered a severe famine. It was noticed by Dutch doctors that patients with coeliac disease improved when there was a shortage of wheat. It led eventually to the discovery that gliadin, a component of wheat, was involved in this disease.

Patients and Controls

The incidence of 'acute anterior uveitis' in HLA-B27-associated ankylosing spondylitis is about 30%. Furthermore, about half of patients with HLA-B27-positive acute anterior uveitis fulfil the criteria of ankylosing spondylitis or reactive arthritis (Linssen et al. 1983). Characteristics of the patients and controls are summarized in the Table 7.1.

The first three groups of patients with acute anterior uveitis had a complete ophthalmological assessment. The patients in the fourth group had ankylosing spondylitis but had never complained of eye problems and therefore were not examined by an ophthalmologist.

The sex ratio was almost equal in the acute anterior uveitis patients who did not have ankylosing spondylitis.

However, in the patients with ankylosing spondylitis, the male/female ratio was about 2/1.

The sex ratio was not determined in the rheumatoid arthritis patients.

The sera from ankylosing spondylitis, acute anterior uveitis and rheumatoid arthritis patients as well as controls were numbered in Amsterdam in such a way that the laboratory in London was not aware of their origin.

The code was broken in Amsterdam after the serological results arrived back from London.

TABLE 7.1 Characteristics of the six groups of patients and the two groups of healthy controls

	AAU only			AS			RA	Controls	
Number of subjects	17	17	17	17	17	17	25	17	17
Male/female	7/10	8/9	11/6	15/2	12/5	ND	8/7	5/7
Mean age (years)	46	44	37	38	44	ND	37	32
Mean ESR (mm/h)	ND	ND	ND	ND	ND	56	ND	ND
Mean CRP (mg/l)	4.9	7.3	11.0	12.0	25.3	25.8	5.9	4.2
HLA-B27	+	–	+	+	+	ND	+	–
Acute anterior uveitis (AAU)	+	–	+	–	ND	ND	–	–

Due to identity protection, sex and age were not known for some controls

ESR erythrocyte sedimentation rate, CRP C-reactive protein, AS ankylosing spondylitis, ND not done

Serum C-Reactive Protein Levels

Serum C-reactive protein levels were measured by the single radial immunodiffusion method of Mancini.

Serum C-reactive protein levels in the two control groups were relatively low (Table 7.1).

Serum C-reactive protein levels were found to be highest in HLA-B27-positive patients with active ankylosing spondylitis and patients with active rheumatoid arthritis when compared to all other disease groups or controls.

Of the remainder, only two groups showed any significant elevation in C-reactive protein levels. The HLA-B27-positive, acute anterior uveitis–positive, ankylosing spondylitis–positive patients had higher levels of C-reactive protein when compared to HLA-B27-positive controls ($t = 1.60$, $p < 0.05$). The other group consisted of HLA-B27-positive, acute anterior uveitis–negative, ankylosing spondylitis–positive patients who also had an elevated level of C-reactive protein ($t = 2.14$, $p < 0.025$). Furthermore, HLA-B27-positive, acute anterior uveitis–positive, ankylosing spondylitis patients had a higher level of C-reactive protein when compared to HLA-B27-negative controls ($t = 2.02$, $p < 2.60$). A similar significant elevation in C-reactive protein level was observed in the HLA-B27-positive, acute anterior uveitis–negative, ankylosing spondylitis–positive patients when compared to the HLA-B27-negative controls ($t = 2.60$, $p < 0.005$).

Indirect Immunofluorescence Studies with *Proteus* and *Klebsiella* in Rheumatoid Arthritis, Ankylosing Spondylitis and Acute Anterior Uveitis Patients from the Netherlands

Indirect immunofluorescence assay was carried out as previously described.

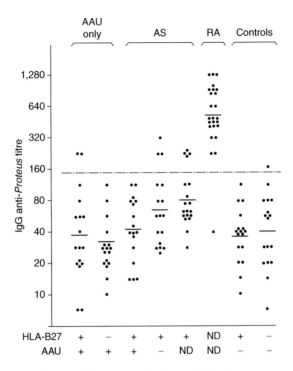

FIGURE 7.1 IgG anti-*Proteus mirabilis* antibody titres in sera of patients from groups 1–8 (Table 7.1). Each *dot* represents either a control subject or a patient (With permission from Blankenberg-Sprenkels et al. (1998))

IgG Antibodies to Proteus mirabilis

Patients with active rheumatoid arthritis patients showed significant elevations in IgG antibody titre when compared to either HLA-B27-positive controls ($t = 12.3$, $p < 001$) or when compared to HLA-B27-negative controls ($t = 10.6$, $p < 0.001$) (Fig. 7.1).

This antibody elevation in anti-*Proteus* titre was also significant when compared to all the other groups: HLA-B27-positive, acute anterior uveitis–positive, ankylosing spondylitis–positive patients ($t=10.8$, $p<0.001$), HLA-B27-positive, acute anterior uveitis–positive, ankylosing spondylitis–negative patients ($t=9.79$, $p<0.001$), HLA-B27-positive, acute anterior uveitis–negative, ankylosing spondylitis–positive patients ($t=8.6$, $p<0.001$) and HLA-B27-positive patients with active ankylosing spondylitis ($t=8.8$, $p<0.001$).

IgA Antibodies to Klebsiella pneumoniae

HLA-B27 positive patients with active ankylosing spondylitis showed the highest levels of IgA antibodies to *Klebsiella pneumoniae* and this was significantly higher than in HLA-B27-positive healthy controls ($t=6.27$, $p<0.001$) or HLA-B27-negative healthy controls ($t=11.37$, $p<0.001$) or in patients with rheumatoid arthritis ($t=11.36$, $p<0.001$) (Fig. 7.2).

Although no other ankylosing spondylitis or acute anterior uveitis showed anti-*Klebsiella* antibody titres above that of the patients with active ankylosing spondylitis, there were elevations above those seen in controls and patients with rheumatoid arthritis.

Patients who were HLA-B27-positive, acute anterior uveitis–positive and ankylosing spondylitis–positive and those who were HLA-B27-positive, acute anterior uveitis–negative and ankylosing spondylitis–positive had higher anti-*Klebsiella* antibody titres than patients who were HLA-B27-positive, anterior uveitis–positive, ankylosing spondylitis–negative but these differences were not statistically significant when corrected for number of groups examined. The titre of anti-*Klebsiella* antibodies could not be related to exacerbations or remissions in patients with acute anterior uveitis.

Furthermore HLA-B27-negative, acute anterior uveitis–positive and ankylosing spondylitis–negative patients had higher titres of anti-*Klebsiella* antibodies than either HLA-B27-positive controls ($t=2.16$, $p<0.05$) or HLA-B27-negative controls ($t=6.37$, $p<0.001$).

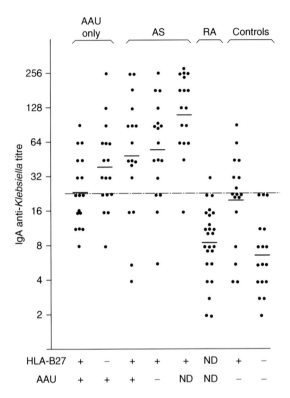

FIGURE 7.2 IgA anti-*Klebsiella pneumoniae* antibody titres in sera of patients from groups 1–8 (Table 7.1). Each *dot* represents either a control subject or a patient (With permission from Blankenberg-Sprenkels et al. (1998))

Clinical Implications

Rheumatoid arthritis patients had antibodies to *Proteus*, and ankylosing spondylitis and acute anterior uveitis patients had antibodies to *Klebsiella*. Each disease group was a specificity control for the other condition. It is clear that rheumatoid arthritis patients had antibodies against *Proteus* but not against

Klebsiella whilst the opposite was observed with the ankylosing spondylitis sera which had antibodies against *Klebsiella* but not against *Proteus.* Professor Bert Feltkamp said he was utterly surprised when his registrar told him that the London studies had picked both groups. The three original centres then refused to re-test the ankylosing spondylitis sera.

Here we are against the problem of simple, commercial test kits not being available to measure anti-*Klebsiella* or anti-*Proteus* antibodies which hampers clinical studies in patients with these diseases. The indirect immunofluorescence assay had been developed in house, in the Immunology Unit of King's College in the University of London by a very capable microbiologist, Dr. Mark Fielder who carried out the assays on the Dutch sera.

These results together with the immunofluorescence data from Toulouse and Brest confirm the previous work from our group in London, the studies from Dublin in Ireland and Newcastle in England that active rheumatoid arthritis patients have antibodies against a urinary pathogen.

An interesting observation was made in the tissue-typed controls. Those subjects who were HLA-B27-positive and deemed clinically healthy showed higher IgA anti-*Klebsiella* antibody titres than those healthy subjects typed as HLA-B27-negative. Similar observations have been made in England (Trull et al. 1983). In Finland, it was found that healthy HLA-B27-positive persons had elevated anti-*Klebsiella* titres of all immunoglobulin classes although only the IgM titres were statistically significantly increased (Toivanen et al. 1993). This may indicate that some subjects in the HLA-B27-positive 'healthy' control group are more likely to develop anti-*Klebsiella* antibodies. The higher anti-*Klebsiella* antibody titre in the HLA-B27 positive control group may also suggest a slow onset of ankylosing spondylitis but only longitudinal studies with close clinical follow-up and regular measurement of antibody levels to *Klebsiella pneumoniae* would resolve the problem.

The interesting question arises whether a similar observation occurs in healthy individuals who carry the 'shared epitope' EQRRAA compared to individuals who are 'shared epitope' negative. Since approximately 35% of the general population in England, USA and the Netherlands carry the 'shared epitope', it would be relevant to determine whether such individuals have raised antibody levels against *Proteus mirabilis*.

If such antibodies are present, then they could act as early markers of rheumatoid arthritis. This would be similar to the situation of anti-CCP antibodies which are known to appear in the early stages of rheumatoid arthritis (Schellekens et al. 1998).

Conclusions

The data presented here show that there are specific and significant antibody elevations against *Proteus mirabilis* in rheumatoid arthritis patients from Amsterdam in the Netherlands. There are no antibody elevations against *Proteus mirabilis* in Dutch patients with acute anterior uveitis or ankylosing spondylitis. However, Dutch patients with ankylosing spondylitis or acute anterior uveitis have specific elevations in antibodies against *Klebsiella* microbes.

References

Blankenberg-Sprenkels SHD, Fielder M, Feltkamp TEW, Tiwana H, Wilson C, Ebringer A. Antibodies to *Klebsiella pneumonia* in Dutch patients with ankylosing spondylitis and acute anterior uveitis and to *Proteus mirabilis* in rheumatoid arthritis. J Rheumatol. 1998; 25:743–7.

Linssen A, Dekker-Saeys AJ, Dandrieu MR, Christiaans BJ, Baarsma GS, Tjoa ST, et al. Possible ankylosing spondylitis in acute anterior uveitis. Br J Rheumatol. 1983;22 Suppl 2:137–43.

Schellekens GA, de Jong BA, van den Hoogen FH, van de Putte LB, van Venrooij WJ. Citrulline is an essential component of antigenic determinants recognized by rheumatoid arthritis specific autoantibodies. J Clin Invest. 1998;101:273–81.

Toivanen P, Koskimies S, Granfors K, Eerola E. Bacterial antibodies in HLA-B27 positive individuals. Arthritis Rheum. 1993;36: 1633–5.

Trull AK, Ebringer R, Panayi GS, Colthorpe D, James DCO, Ebringer A. IgA antibodies to *Klebsiella pneumoniae* in ankylosing spondylitis. Scand J Rheumatol. 1983;12:249–53.

Chapter 8
Anti-*Proteus* Antibodies in Norwegian Rheumatoid Arthritis Patients Following a Lactovegetarian Diet

Contents

Norway: An Introduction

Norway is a Nordic country occupying the western part of the Scandinavian peninsula. It is a country of famous fjords and has a population of about five million.

It was united into one kingdom by Harald the First of Norway in the early 800s which was then followed by two

A. Ebringer, *Rheumatoid Arthritis and Proteus*,
DOI 10.1007/978-0-85729-950-5_8,
© Springer-Verlag London Limited 2012

centuries of Viking raids into various parts of Europe including England, Scotland and Ireland.

Colonies were also established in Iceland, Greenland, North America also known as Vinland and Eastern Europe.

In 1397, it was absorbed into a union with Denmark. Following the destruction of the kingdom of Denmark–Norway during the Napoleonic wars, it merged with Sweden. However, in 1905, following a plebiscite, Norway became an independent country.

It is a country with a high life-expectancy and rheumatoid arthritis is a common disease, as in all countries where there is a high proportion of the population over the age of 50 years.

Patient Population and Diet Study

It has been suggested that *Proteus mirabilis*, a microbe known to cause urinary tract infections, might be relevant in the study of the pathogenesis of rheumatoid arthritis.

A Norwegian group, led by Dr. J. Kjeldsen-Kragh, examined the association between disease activity in rheumatoid arthritis patients during a controlled clinical trial of fasting and a 1-year vegetarian diet (Kjeldsen-Kragh et al. 1991). He had heard about the work in London about antibodies to *Proteus* in rheumatoid arthritis patients and asked us to cooperate in a coded study.

Fasting is an effective method of treating rheumatoid arthritis, but most patients relapse on reintroduction of food.

The effect of fasting followed by 1 year of a vegetarian diet was assessed in a randomised, single-blind control trial. Briefly 53 rheumatoid arthritis patients were studied: 27 rheumatoid arthritis patients were randomly assigned to the diet group and 26 rheumatoid arthritis patients were assigned to the control group. The diet group were invited to a 4-week stay at a health farm. After an initial 7–10 day subtotal fast, they were put on an individually adjusted gluten-free vegan diet for 3.5 months. The food was then gradually changed to a lactovegetarian diet for the remainder of the study. The quantity of fluid intake was not measured.

A control group of 26 rheumatoid arthritis patients stayed for 4 weeks at a convalescent home but ate their ordinary, omnivorous diet throughout the whole study period.

Ten patients were withdrawn from the treatment group and nine from the control group during the course of the study.

After 4 weeks at the health farm, the diet group showed a significant improvement in the number of tender joints, the Ritchie articular index, number of swollen joints, pain score, duration of early morning stiffness, erythrocyte sedimentation rate, C-reactive protein levels, white blood cell count and a health assessment questionnaire score.

In the control group, only the pain assessment score improved.

Blood samples were collected at baseline, and after 1, 4, 7, 10 and 13 months. Serum samples were stored at $-20°C$ until required for analysis.

The rheumatoid arthritis patients in the vegetarian group were subsequently divided into diet responders and diet non-responders, depending on the clinical results following the diet.

Briefly, a rheumatoid arthritis patient was categorised as a diet responder if there had been a substantial improvement in three of six core variables: number of swollen joints, functional disability, pain score, number of tender joints, patient's global assessment and erythrocyte sedimentation rate. The distinction into diet responder and diet non-responder was made before the antibody analyses were carried out.

Antibody analyses against *Proteus mirabilis* and *Escherichia coli* were carried out in all three groups of rheumatoid arthritis patients: diet responders, diet non-responders and controls.

Serum samples were coded in Norway, then sent to the Immunology Unit at King's College in London where the antibody assays were carried out. The results were then sent back to Norway where they were decoded.

In the diet responder group, the benefits were still present after 1 year. The evaluation of the whole course showed significant improvements for the diet in all measured indices.

Disease Activity Index

The relationship between disease activity and the levels of antibodies against *Proteus mirabilis* and *Escherichia coli* was investigated in all rheumatoid arthritis patients. The disease activity at each clinical examination was graded by means of a Stoke disease activity index, slightly modified by replacing the proximal interphalangeal joint synovitis score with the total number of swollen joints (Davis et al. 1990).

Determination of *Proteus mirabilis* and *Escherichia coli* Antibody Titres

ELISA determinations on whole bacteria were carried out as previously described. The statistical analyses were carried out as follows:

To test for within-group differences, the Wilcoxon signed rank test was used. Kruskal–Wallis test was used for comparison of three groups. As a post hoc test for the latter comparisons, the Mann–Whitney test was used. Correlations were studied by Spearman's rank correlation analysis. For the patients who were prematurely withdrawn from the trial, values were extrapolated as described (Kjeldsen-Kragh et al. 1991).

In all tests, except for post hoc analyses, p-values less than 0.05 were considered as significant.

As the post hoc analyses involved three comparisons, only those p-values less than 0.0167 were regarded as significant for these tests.

Results of the Antibody Assays in Rheumatoid Arthritis Patients

Patients who followed the lactovegetarian diet had a significant reduction in mean anti-*Proteus* antibody titre at 4, 7, 10 and 13 months (Table 8.1).

TABLE 8.1 Decrease from baseline with time for anti-*Proteus mirabilis* and anti-*Escherichia coli* IgG ($\log_2$ dilution units). Statistical significance compared to baseline

| | Time elapsed after baseline measurements | | |
	7 months	10 months	13 months
Anti-*Proteus* antibody	$p < 0.01$	$p < 0.01$	$p < 0.01$
Diet responders	1.417	1.125	1.042
Diet non-responders	0.467	0.200	0.233
Omnivores	−0.077	0.346	0.385
Anti-*E.coli* antibody	NS	NS	NS
Diet responders	0.058	0.025	0.089
Diet non-responders	−0.035	−0.073	−0.062
Omnivores	0.004	−0.006	−0.013

NS not significant

No significant change in mean antibody titre was observed in the omnivorous patients.

In the rheumatoid arthritis patients who eventually were categorised as 'diet responders', the mean anti-*Proteus* antibody titre decreased significantly compared with baseline after 1, 4, 7 and 10 months. At all these times, the antibody titres were least for the diet responders; post hoc analysis revealed that the change from baseline was significantly greater in the diet responders compared to the rheumatoid arthritis patients in the control, omnivorous group.

Changes from baseline of the modified Stoke disease activity index were examined with the changes from baseline with the anti-*Proteus mirabilis* and the anti-*Escherichia coli* antibody levels.

Disease improvement correlated significantly with the anti-Proteus *mirabilis* titres ($r = 0.31$, $p < 0.001$) (Fig. 8.1) but not with the changes in anti-*Escherichia coli* antibody levels ($r = -0.012$, not significant).

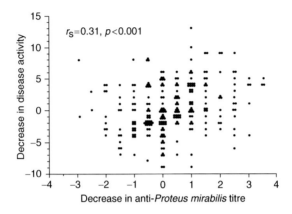

FIGURE 8.1 Scattergram of the decrease from baseline in anti-*Proteus* titres in the rheumatoid arthritis patients versus the decrease from baseline in the modified Stoke disease activity index. *p*-value by Spearman rank correlation (r_s=correlation coefficient) (Reprinted from Kjeldsen-Kragh et al. (1995), with permission from BMJ Publishing Group)

The lack of a significant correlation with anti-*Escherichia coli* antibodies in Norwegian patients with rheumatoid arthritis is in agreement with the studies on Bermudian and English patients from Stevenage with rheumatoid arthritis who also showed no association with the cystitis causing bladder microbe, namely *Escherichia coli.*

All statistical analyses were also performed on the original data that had not been extrapolated to account for withdrawn patients. These analyses gave almost the same results as the analyses for the extrapolated data.

Discussion

This is a comprehensive longitudinal study of anti-*Proteus mirabilis* antibodies in rheumatoid arthritis patients following dietary therapy. A significant decrease in anti-*Proteus mirabilis* antibodies was found in the diet responders compared with the diet non-responders and omnivores (Kjeldsen-Kragh et al. 1995).

The decrease in *Proteus* antibody titres further substantiates the suggestion that these antibodies are of central importance in the pathogenesis of rheumatoid arthritis.

Fasting and vegetarian diets give rise to significant changes in the gastro-intestinal bacterial flora (Midvedt et al. 1990). Furthermore, uncooked vegan diets alter the microbial bowel flora (Peltonen et al. 1992).

Peltonen's group have analysed the faecal flora collected from rheumatoid arthritis patients who participated in the controlled clinical trial of fasting and 1-year vegetarian diet (Peltonen et al. 1994).

Significant differences in the faecal flora were observed between samples obtained at times which coincided with pronounced clinical improvement and samples obtained at times of low or no improvement. However, it remains to be demonstrated that these differences were the result of a decrease in the amount of *Proteus mirabilis* in the faeces, which in turn might reduce the absorption of *Proteus* antigens from the gut.

A shift from an omnivorous diet to a vegetarian diet has a profound influence on the composition of the urine. Vegetarians may have an increased fluid intake although this was not specifically investigated in this study. High fluid intake has been thought to be beneficial in patients with urinary tract infections and this could explain the decreased anti-*Proteus mirabilis* antibody titres in rheumatoid arthritis patients on lactovegetarian diets. Furthermore, some plant products like cranberry juice are frequently used in the treatment of urinary tract infections.

Vegetarians have a greater urinary excretion of lignans and phytooestrogens metabolites than omnivores. Some of these substances are known to possess antibacterial activity in vitro (Ito et al. 1982).

A positive correlation between C-reactive protein levels and the level of anti-*Proteus* antibody titres has been reported by the London group and the Newcastle group.

In the present study, a significant correlation was found between the changes in anti-*Proteus* antibody titres and the changes in a disease activity index composed of five different variables following a lactovegetarian diet. Clearly further studies are indicated to determine the role of anti-*Proteus* antibodies in the pathogenesis of rheumatoid arthritis.

References

Davis MJ, Dawes PT, Fowler PD, Sheeran TP, Shadforth MF, Ziade F, et al. Comparison and evaluation of disease activity index for use in patients with rheumatoid arthritis. Br J Rheumatol. 1990;29: 111–5.

Ito K, Iida T, Ichino K, Tsunezuka M, Hattori M, Namba T. Obovatol and obovatal, novel biphenyl ether lignans from the leaves of Magnoliaobovata Thunb. Chem Pharm Bull. 1982;30:791–7.

Kjeldsen-Kragh J, Haugen M, Borchgrevink C, Laerum E, Eek M, Mowinkel P, et al. Controlled trial of fasting and one year vegetarian diet in rheumatoid arthritis. Lancet. 1991;338:889–902.

Kjeldsen-Kragh J, Rashid T, Dybwad A, Sioud M, Haugen M, Forre O, et al. Decrease in anti-*Proteus mirabilis* but not anti-*Escherichia coli* antibody levels in rheumatoid arthritis patients treated with fasting and a one year vegetarian diet. Ann Rheum Dis. 1995;54:221–4.

Midvedt T, Johansson G, Carlstedt-Duke B, Midvedt A-C, Norin KE, Gustafsson JA. The effect of a shift from a mixed to a lacto-vegetarian diet on some intestinal microflora associated characteristics. Microb Ecol Health Dis. 1990;3:33–8.

Peltonen R, Ling W-H, Hänninen O, Eerola E. An uncooked vegan diet shifts the profile of human fecal microflora: computerised analysis of direct stool sample gas-liquid chromatography profiles of bacterial cellular fatty acids. Appl Environ Microbiol. 1992;58:3660–6.

Peltonen R, Kjeldsen-Kragh J, Haugen M, Tuominen J, Toivanen P, Forre O, et al. Changes in fecal flora in rheumatoid arthritis patients during fasting and one year vegetarian diet. Br J Rheumatol. 1994;33:638–43.

Chapter 9
Antibodies to *Proteus* in Rheumatoid Arthritis Patients from Norway, Spain and England

Contents

A. Ebringer, *Rheumatoid Arthritis and Proteus*,
DOI 10.1007/978-0-85729-950-5_9,
© Springer-Verlag London Limited 2012

Norway, Spain and Epsom in England: An Introduction

In the early 1990s, an industrious and enthusiastic student from Spain, Mr. A. Marti, came to King's College to study biological sciences under a European Common Market Studentship. When he heard that our research interest involved investigating patients with rheumatoid arthritis, he said that physicians in his native town, Barcelona in Catalonia, a rich and industrial part of Spain, would be very agreeable to carry out a joint study. He introduced us to Dr. Antonio Collado from the Department of Rheumatology in the Hospital Clinic i Provincial de Barcelona who agreed to participate in a three-country study of rheumatoid arthritis patients.

Rheumatoid arthritis patients from three different countries of Europe, Norway, Spain and England, would be tested simultaneously against controls from their respective countries under blind conditions by research workers in the Immunology Unit of the Division of Life Sciences at King's College in London.

The two other groups, one from Norway and the other one from Epsom in Surrey, England, had shown that exacerbations in disease activity in rheumatoid arthritis patients could be modified by careful attention to environmental parameters such as diet, fluid intake and exercise. Furthermore we had shown that Norwegian rheumatoid arthritis patients treated with fasting and a lacto-vegetarian diet showed a decrease in anti-*Proteus* antibodies if they were deemed to have clinically improved and labelled as 'diet-responders'.

Clinicians in the three countries were interested in our investigations into the origin of rheumatoid arthritis and provided samples from their rheumatoid arthritis patients as well as controls for this study.

It was decided to compare Catalan patients from Barcelona with Norwegian rheumatoid arthritis patients as well as a group of English rheumatoid arthritis patients attending the Department of Rheumatology of the Epsom General Hospital in Surrey, in England under the care of Dr. Gail Darlington.

Dr. Darlington had been investigating for several years dietary trigger factors in rheumatoid arthritis patients (Darlington et al. 1986).

Oslo: Location and History

Oslo is the capital and largest city in Norway. It is located in the southern part of the country on the Oslofjord. It was founded in 1048 by King Harald III of Norway. The city was largely destroyed by fire in 1624.

It has a population of about one and half million. The Munch Museum opened in 1963. Over the last decades, Norway and Oslo have become very prosperous and it is not surprising that it is one of the most expensive cities in the world.

The Sanitetsforening Rheumatism Hospital is located in Oslo and the rheumatoid arthritis patients came from Prof. O. Forre's Department of Rheumatology.

Barcelona: Location and History

Barcelona is located in the north-eastern region of the Iberian peninsula and is the second largest town in Spain after Madrid.

In 218 B.C. at the start of the second Punic War, it was occupied by Carthaginian troops under Hamilcar Barca. This military occupation is often cited as the foundation of the modern city of Barcelona.

Subsequently, it was occupied by the Romans, Visigoths, then Moslems and finally it was captured by the son of Charlemagne, Louis the Pious.

During the Middle Ages, it was part of the Kingdom of Aragon.

Barcelona suffered greatly during the Spanish Civil War and this is well described by George Orwell in his book 'Homage to Catalonia'. Because of its resistance to the Franco regime, the use of the Catalan language was forbidden for many years.

Barcelona has a population of about one and half million and has many architectural buildings, such as the unfinished 'Familia Sagrada' designed by Antoni Gaudi.

Dr. Antonio Collado from the Hospital Clinic I Provincial de Barcelona provided serum samples obtained from Spanish rheumatoid arthritis subjects.

Epsom in Surrey

The town of Epsom is located just south-west of London. Epsom appears in the Domesday Book 1086, but over the years, it has become part of the London conurbation.

Dr. Gail Darlington from the Epsom General Hospital provided serum samples from her rheumatoid arthritis patients.

Patients and Controls

Rheumatoid arthritis has been the subject of more population studies than any other rheumatic disease and the most striking feature is the overall similarity in prevalence between populations, with a standard rate of between 0.5% and 1% (Silman 1993). This consistency is most unusual in human chronic diseases and may reflect the ubiquity of the causative factors whether genetic and/or environmental.

The possibility that rheumatoid arthritis has an infectious aetiology has spurred attempts to identify such agents. Early attempts were made to suggest that rheumatoid arthritis may have a link with *Streptococcus* infection (Cecil et al. 1930).

More recently, a possible association with the urinary microbe *Proteus mirabilis* has been proposed based on molecular mimicry studies and immunological investigations in several countries.

In an endeavour to test the geographical consistency of these observations, rheumatoid arthritis patients from three different countries, Epsom in England, Oslo in Norway and

Barcelona from Spain, were compared to determine the involvement of the microbe *Proteus mirabilis* in rheumatoid arthritis.

A total of 114 serum samples were collected from rheumatoid arthritis patients in Norway, Spain and England, and tested for IgG anti-*Proteus* antibodies by the indirect immunofluorescence technique.

A group of 27 English rheumatoid arthritis patients were recruited from the Rheumatology Clinics at the Epsom District Hospital, Surrey, 34 Spanish rheumatoid arthritis patients were recruited from the Rheumatology Department, Hospital Clinic I Provincial in Barcelona while the third group consisted of 53 Norwegian rheumatoid arthritis patients attending the Outpatient department of the Oslo Sanitetsforenings Rheumatism Hospital in Oslo. All these patients were diagnosed according to the revised American College of Rheumatology criteria (Arnett et al. 1988).

The rheumatoid arthritis patient groups were generally classified into those with an either active disease or inactive disease. Active disease patients were defined biochemically as those having a C-reactive protein level equal or above 10 mg/l. Inactive disease patients were those having a C-reactive protein level below 10 mg/l. Active and inactive disease groups were then analysed separately for each country.

Serum samples from a group of 30 Norwegian, 14 Spanish and 25 English healthy controls were collected and also screened for anti-*Proteus* antibody titres. None of these control individuals had a history of acute or chronic rheumatic disease.

Indirect Immunofluorescence Studies

Indirect immunofluorescence studies were carried out as previously described.

The difference in the mean antibody titre between two groups was compared using Student's *t*-test. The relationship

TABLE 9.1 General characteristics and serum C-reactive protein levels (mg/l) in rheumatoid arthritis (RA) and healthy controls (HC) among the three populations studied

| | Populations studied | | | | | |
| | English | | Norwegian | | Spanish | |
	RA	HC	RA	HC	RA	HC
Number of subjects	27	25	53	30	34	14
Age (years)						
Mean	50.6	25.8	53.0	47.0	56.4	53.0
Range	30–76	22–36	26–78	28–77	26–8	33–64
Sex						
Males	7	10	8	4	12	6
Females	20	15	45	26	22	8
C-reactive protein (mg/l)	14.8	2.1	13.3	4.0	16.8	1.6
	$p < 0.005$		$p < 0.001$		$p < 0.005$	

between anti-*Proteus* antibody titre and C-reactive protein levels in the tested sera was estimated using Spearman's rank correlation coefficient.

General Characteristics of the Groups and Analysis of the C-Reactive Protein Levels

The mean age and range as well as sex distribution of rheumatoid arthritis patients and healthy controls from each population were approximately comparable to each other (Table 9.1).

The mean ± standard error of serum C-reactive protein levels was significantly higher ($t = 9.27$, $p < 0.005$) in English rheumatoid arthritis patients (14.8 ± 3.4 mg/l) when compared to English controls (2.1 ± 1.7 mg/l).

The mean ± standard error of serum C-reactive protein levels was significantly higher ($t = 9.88, p < 0.001$) in Norwegian rheumatoid arthritis patients (13.3 ± 1.8 mg/l) when compared to Norwegian controls (4.0 ± 0.7 mg/l).

The mean ± standard error of serum C-reactive protein levels was significantly higher ($t = 2.78, p < 0.005$) in Spanish rheumatoid arthritis patients (16.8 ± 3.5 mg/l) when compared to Spanish controls (1.6 ± 0.2 mg/l).

However, no such significant difference in mean C-reactive protein level was observed when the English rheumatoid arthritis group was compared with the Spanish or Norwegian patients. Also there was no significant difference in serum C-reactive protein levels between the Spanish and Norwegian rheumatoid arthritis groups.

Anti-*Proteus* Antibodies in Active and Inactive Rheumatoid Arthritis Patients Compared to Healthy Controls

When the results were analysed according to disease activity as specified by serum C-reactive levels, the active group of rheumatoid arthritis patients showed a significantly higher level of anti-*Proteus* than its corresponding healthy controls, whether this group came from English ($t = 11.42, p < 0.001$), Norwegian ($t = 8.86, p < 0.001$) or Spanish ($t = 5.35, p < 0.001$) populations (Fig. 9.1).

A similar result was observed when the active group of rheumatoid arthritis patients was compared with its counterpart of inactive rheumatoid arthritis patients, whether this group came from English ($t = 9.04, p < 0.01$), Norwegian ($t = 5.48, p < 0.001$) or Spanish ($t = 4.00, p < 0.001$) populations (Fig. 9.1).

A significant elevation in the IgG anti-*Proteus* antibody level was only observed among English inactive rheumatoid arthritis patients ($t = 8.92, p < 0.001$) and Norwegian inactive rheumatoid arthritis patients ($t = 3.49, p < 0.001$) but not Spanish inactive rheumatoid arthritis patients ($t = 0.35$, not significant) when compared to their corresponding healthy subjects.

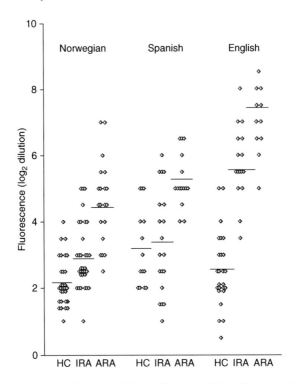

FIGURE 9.1 Anti-*Proteus* IgG (log$_2$ dilution units) antibody levels in sera of active (*ARA*) and inactive (*IRA*) rheumatoid arthritis patients and healthy controls (*HC*) in Norwegian, Spanish and English populations (Reprinted with permission from Rashid et al. (1999))

Correlation of Serum C-Reactive Protein Levels with Anti-*Proteus* Antibodies

When the serum C-reactive protein level was compared with the anti-*Proteus* antibody titre in the sera of all rheumatoid arthritis patients within the English, Norwegian and Spanish populations, there was a significant positive correlation between these two variables ($r = +0.47$, $p < 0.0001$) (Fig. 9.2).

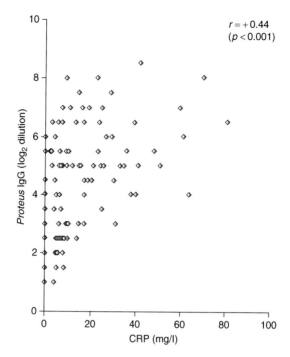

FIGURE 9.2 Correlation analysis between levels of anti-*Proteus* IgG antibodies and C-reactive protein (*CRP*) levels in the sera of Norwegian, Spanish and English patients with rheumatoid arthritis ($n = 114$) (Reprinted with permission from Rashid et al. (1999))

The correlation coefficients were also significant when the Norwegian ($r = +0.53, p < 0.001$), English ($r = +0.70, p < 0.0005$) and Spanish ($r = +0.62$) populations were analysed separately.

Disease Activity and Conclusions

These simultaneous results from three different European countries support the observations made previously in London, Dublin, Bermuda and France.

Antibody levels to *Proteus* bacteria are consistently elevated in patients with rheumatoid arthritis especially during active phases of inflammation, as defined by increased serum C-reactive protein levels, when compared to healthy individuals.

The presence of elevated anti-*Proteus* antibodies in rheumatoid arthritis patients would appear to be linked to active phases of inflammation and is not part of the phenotype of the disease. Therefore, when looking for aetiological factors, disease activity should not be defined by clinical criteria but by biochemical criteria such as C-reactive protein levels or elevated erythrocyte sedimentation rate. A rheumatoid arthritis patient having many joint deformities but having no evidence of inflammatory disease at the point in time when a blood sample is obtained, as defined by C-reactive protein levels or erythrocyte sedimentation rates, would not be expected to have elevated levels of anti-*Proteus* antibodies. This is an important distinction in the study of the aetiology of this disease.

The correlation with C-reactive protein would appear to indicate that there is an immunological process involving the binding of antibodies to tissue components such as HLA molecules with subsequent stimulation of interleukins (Ganapathi et al. 1991).

In this standardised indirect immunofluorescence assay, the whole *Proteus* microbe was used, instead of degraded bacterial particles so as to recognise as much of the antigenic profile as possible.

The specificity of response was investigated by the Newcastle group who could not observe any significant correlation between antibody levels against *Proteus mirabilis* and antibody titres against four viruses, influenza, adenovirus, rubella and parvovirus (Deighton et al. 1992).

Furthermore, the same group could not find any correlation between the anti-*Proteus* antibody titre and eight autoantibodies: rheumatoid factor, thyroglobulin, thyroid microsomal, antinuclear, parietal cell, mitochondrial, smooth muscle and reticulin antibodies.

In conclusion, increased levels of anti-*Proteus* antibodies in rheumatoid arthritis patients from three different countries confirm the geographical if not the worldwide consistency of this observation and support the likelihood that this microbe is involved in the aetiopathogenesis of this disease (Rashid et al. 1999).

References

Arnett F, Edworthy S, Bloch D, McShane D, Fries J, Cooper N, et al. The American Rheumatism Association 1987 revised criteria for the classification of rheumatoid arthritis. Arthritis Rheum. 1988;31:315–24.

Cecil R, Nicholls E, Stansby W. Characteristics of *Streptococci* isolated from patients with rheumatic fever and chronic infectious arthritis. Am J Pathol. 1930;6:619–25.

Darlington G, Ramsey N, Mansfield J. Placebo controlled, blind study of dietary manipulation therapy in rheumatoid arthritis. Lancet. 1986;1:236–8.

Deighton CM, Gray J, Bint AJ, Walker DJ. Specificity of the *Proteus* antibody response in rheumatoid arthritis. Ann Rheum Dis. 1992;51:1206–7.

Ganapathi M, Rzewnicki D, Samols D, Jiang S, Kushner I. Effect of combination of cytokines and hormones on synthesis of serum amyloid A and C-reactive protein in HEP 3B cells. J Immunol. 1991;147:1261–5.

Rashid T, Darlington G, Kjeldsen-Kragh FO, Collado A, Ebringer A. *Proteus* IgG antibodies and C-reactive protein in English, Norwegian and Spanish patients with rheumatoid arthritis. Clin Rheumatol. 1999;18:190–5.

Silman A. Epidemiology and the rheumatic diseases. In: Maddison P, Isenberg D, Woo P, editors. Oxford textbook of rheumatology. Oxford: Oxford University Press; 1993. p. 499–513.

Chapter 10
Antibodies to *Proteus* in Rheumatoid Arthritis Patients from Southern Japan

Contents

The Japanese Connection: An Introduction

In the early 1980s, the Immunology Unit of King's College had shown that there were elevated levels of antibodies to the Gram-negative bowel microbe *Klebsiella* in patients suffering from ankylosing spondylitis. These patients were being investigated in the 'Ankylosing Spondylitis Research Unit' of the Middlesex Hospital which had been set up in 1976 to study why up to 96% of ankylosing spondylitis with this disease possessed the HLA-B27 Major Histocompatibility group antigen whilst the frequency of this antigen in the general population of England or of the USA was only 8%.

A. Ebringer, *Rheumatoid Arthritis and Proteus*,
DOI 10.1007/978-0-85729-950-5_10,
© Springer-Verlag London Limited 2012

However, immunological studies in Japan showed that HLA-B27 was present in only 0.4% of the Japanese population, one of the lowest frequencies throughout the world.

Furthermore, ankylosing spondylitis, as a disease, was extremely rare in Japan, so rare that when the disease was observed, it was referred to orthopaedic surgeons because of their interests in backache and not to rheumatologists.

In 1993, I was approached by Professor Sinsuke Hukuda from Shiga University that a promising research worker and orthopaedic surgeon Dr. Yoshitaka Tani had been awarded a visiting scholarship from the Rheumatism Foundation of Japan to come to London and study antibodies to *Klebsiella* in Japanese ankylosing spondylitis patients. Since ankylosing spondylitis belonged to the orthopaedic medical community in Japan because of its rarity, it attracted the attention of this ambitious and hard working orthopaedic surgeon, Dr. Yoshitaka Tani as a research project. He collected all the ankylosing spondylitis patients in the southern parts of Japan and decided to determine whether they had elevated levels of antibodies to *Klebsiella* as had been reported in ankylosing spondylitis patients in England (Trull et al. 1983).

Dr. Yoshitaka Tani came to London with his ankylosing spondylitis sera and blood donor control sera. The ankylosing spondylitis and control sera were stored in a freezer, and he was told he should go back to Japan and bring back as well sera from active rheumatoid arthritis patients.

Active rheumatoid arthritis patients were defined as those having at least an erythrocyte sedimentation rate in excess of 30 mm/h (ESR > 30 mm/h) at the time when the blood sample was obtained. Then both ankylosing spondylitis sera and rheumatoid arthritis sera would be tested simultaneously against both *Klebsiella* and *Proteus* bacteria, under blind conditions in London. Each microbe would be acting as a disease control for the other condition.

Dr. Yoshitaka Tani returned to Japan and brought back to London a set of sera obtained from Japanese active rheumatoid arthritis patients from the Otsu area in southern Japan.

All the sera, from rheumatoid arthritis and ankylosing spondylitis patients as well as from the blood donors, were then tested under blind conditions against both *Klebsiella* and *Proteus* microorganisms, as well as against *Escherichia coli*.

Otsu: Location and History

Otsu is the capital city of the Shiga province in southern Japan. In 2006, Shiga was merged with Otsu and the size of the merged population was approximately 350,000.

In the years 667–672, Omiotsu Palace was founded in Otsu by Emperor Tenji. During the Edo period (1603–1867) when the Tokugawa shoguns were rulers of Japan, the poet Matsuo Basho frequented Otsu and took on apprentices.

On 11th May 1891, the 'Otsu incident' occurred, during a failed assassination attempt on Tsarevich Nicholas Alexandrovich of Russia.

The Shiga University is in the Shiga Prefecture of Japan. It comprises campuses from the cities of Otsu and Hikone.

The rheumatoid arthritis and ankylosing spondylitis patients came from the Shiga province in Japan.

Patients and Controls

Serum samples from 152 Japanese subjects were studied.

There were 30 patients with active rheumatoid arthritis as defined by the American Rheumatism Association criteria. There were 5 men and 25 women. The female to male ratio was 5:1. The mean age of the active rheumatoid arthritis patients was 51 years (range 23–70 years). The mean (±standard error) erythrocyte sedimentation rate of the active rheumatoid arthritis was 77.7 ± 5.9 mm/h. The mean C-reactive protein level of the active rheumatoid arthritis patients' mean (±standard error) was 40.2 ± 5.2 mg/l.

There were also 20 rheumatoid arthritis patients with probably active disease, 5 men and 15 women. The female to male ratio was 3:1. The mean age of the probably active rheumatoid arthritis patients was 55 years (range 30–77 years). The mean (±standard error) erythrocyte sedimentation rate of the probably active rheumatoid arthritis patients was 38.3±9.4 mm/h. The mean (±standard error) C-reactive protein level of the probably active rheumatoid arthritis patients was 5.9±1.3 mg/l.

There were 29 sera from active ankylosing spondylitis patients selected according to the New York criteria. There were 27 men and 2 women and the male to female ratio was 13.5:1. The mean age of the active ankylosing spondylitis patients was 42 years (range 20–69 years). The mean (±standard error) erythrocyte sedimentation rate of the active ankylosing spondylitis patients was 49.0±9.7 mm/h. The mean (±standard error) C-reactive protein level of the active ankylosing spondylitis patients was 24.8±9.1 mg/l.

There were also 23 ankylosing spondylitis patients with inactive disease (21 men and 2 women) and the male to female ratio was 10.5:1.

The mean age of the inactive ankylosing spondylitis patients was 42 years (range 25–68 years). The mean (±standard error) erythrocyte sedimentation rate of the inactive ankylosing spondylitis was 12.2±2.1 mm/h. The mean (±standard error) C-reactive protein level of the inactive ankylosing spondylitis patients was 3.9±1.1 mg/l.

Furthermore, sera from 50 healthy controls (25 men and 25 women) were supplied by the Red Cross Blood Centre in Otsu, Japan.

Active patients were deemed to be those who had an erythrocyte sedimentation rate greater than 20 mm/h and a serum C-reactive protein level above 10 mg/l.

Probably active patients were considered those with at least one of these variables elevated.

Inactive patients were those with an erythrocyte sedimentation rate below 15 mm/h and a serum C-reactive protein level below 10 mg/l.

All ankylosing spondylitis patients except one were HLA-B27 positive.

Some 93.3% of the active rheumatoid arthritis patients possessed either HLA-DR1 or HLA-DR4. Furthermore, some 40% of the rheumatoid arthritis patients had both HLA-DR1 and DR4.

Control subjects were not tissue typed.

Results of ELISA Studies

ELISA studies were carried out as previously described against three different microbes: *Proteus mirabilis*, *Escherichia coli* and *Klebsiella pneumoniae*. All assays were carried out under code so that the status of each serum sample under investigation was not known to the tester.

Patients with active rheumatoid arthritis showed elevated levels of IgG antibodies against *Proteus mirabilis* when compared to controls and this difference was statistically significant ($t = 14.10, p < 0.001$) (Fig. 10.1).

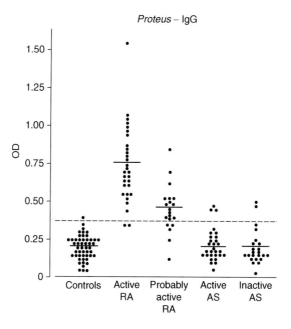

FIGURE 10.1 IgG antibody titres against *Proteus mirabilis* in controls, active rheumatoid arthritis patients, probably active rheumatoid arthritis patients, active ankylosing spondylitis patients and inactive ankylosing spondylitis patients. The *broken line* represents 95% confidence limit of the distribution of the controls (bars = means). Each *dot* represents either a control subject or a patient (Reprinted from Tani et al. (1997), with kind permission)

Similar results were seen in probably active rheumatoid arthritis patients when compared to controls, and this difference was also statistically significant ($t = 8.30, p < 0.001$).

Active rheumatoid arthritis patients also had elevated levels of IgM antibodies against *Proteus mirabilis* when compared to controls and again this difference was statistically significant ($t = 3.72, p < 0.001$).

Probably active rheumatoid arthritis patients did not exhibit IgM antibody elevations against *Proteus mirabilis*.

There were no IgG, IgA or IgM antibody elevations in active or probably active rheumatoid arthritis patients when tested with *Klebsiella pneumoniae* or *Escherichia coli*.

Ankylosing spondylitis patients with active disease had elevated levels of IgA antibodies against *Klebsiella pneumoniae* and this difference was statistically significant when compared to controls ($t = 5.72, p < 0.001$) (Fig. 10.2).

Inactive ankylosing spondylitis patients showed no elevations in IgA, IgG or IgM antibodies against *Klebsiella pneumoniae*.

Active and inactive ankylosing spondylitis had no elevations in IgG or IgM antibodies against *Klebsiella pneumoniae*.

There were no IgG, IgA or IgM antibody elevations in either active or inactive ankylosing spondylitis patients against *Proteus mirabilis* or *Escherichia coli*.

Discussion and Conclusions

The data presented here show that there are specific and significant antibody elevations against *Proteus mirabilis* in rheumatoid arthritis patients from Otsu in southern Japan.

These results would appear to be specific, since Japanese ankylosing spondylitis had antibody elevations against *Klebsiella pneumoniae* but not against *Proteus mirabilis* whilst the reverse was observed with Japanese rheumatoid arthritis patients.

This would appear to be the first time that Japanese rheumatoid arthritis patients have been found to have elevated levels of specific antibodies against the urinary microbe *Proteus mirabilis* (Tani et al. 1997).

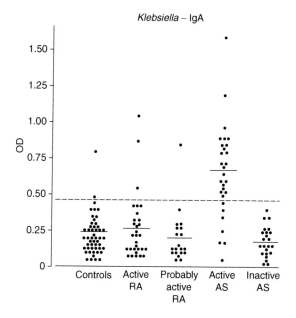

FIGURE 10.2 IgA antibody titres against *Klebsiella pneumoniae* in controls, active rheumatoid arthritis patients, probably active rheumatoid arthritis patients, active ankylosing spondylitis patients and inactive ankylosing spondylitis patients. The *broken line* represents 95% confidence limit of the distribution of the controls (bars = means). Each *dot* represents either a control subject or a patient (Reprinted from Tani et al. (1997), with kind permission)

However, similar Japanese studies have shown that antibodies to 'common enterobacterial antigens' are present in the serum and synovial fluids of patients with rheumatoid arthritis (Aoki et al. 1996).

These results would seem to suggest that the Gram-negative microbe *Proteus mirabilis* is somehow involved in the onset and pathogenesis of rheumatoid arthritis at least in Japanese patients coming from Otsu and surrounding areas. Studies from the USA and Canada indicate that antibodies to

Proteus mirabilis can be detected in the early stages of rheumatoid arthritis (Newkirk et al. 2005).

The results from these Japanese patients appear to be similar to those obtained from rheumatoid arthritis studies in European and American patients.

The general tentative conclusion can be proposed that *Proteus mirabilis* is involved in the causation of rheumatoid arthritis in populations throughout the world.

References

Aoki S, Yoshikawa K, Yokoyama T, Nonogaki T, Wasaki S, Mitsui T, et al. Role of enteric bacteria in the pathogenesis of rheumatoid arthritis: evidence for antibodies to enterobacterial common antigens in rheumatoid sera and synovial fluids. Ann Rheum Dis. 1996;55:363–9.

Newkirk MM, Goldbach-Mansky R, Senior BW, Klippel J, Schumacher HR, El-Gabalawy HS. Elevated levels of IgM and IgA antibodies to *Proteus mirabilis* and IgM antibodies to *Escherichia coli* are associated with early rheumatoid factor (RF)-positive rheumatoid arthritis. Rheumatology. 2005;44:1433–41.

Tani Y, Tiwana H, Hukuda S, Nishioka J, Fielder M, Wilson C, et al. Antibodies to *Klebsiella*, *Proteus* and HLA-B27 peptides in Japanese patients with ankylosing spondylitis and rheumatoid arthritis. J Rheumatol. 1997;24:109–14.

Trull AK, Ebringer R, Panayi GS, Colthorpe D, James DCO, Ebringer A. IgA antibodies to *Klebsiella pneumoniae* in ankylosing spondylitis. Scand J Rheumatol. 1983;12:249–53.

Chapter 11
Urine Cultures and Correlation

Contents

Introduction: Urine Cultures in Rheumatoid Arthritis

Antibodies to *Proteus mirabilis* in rheumatoid arthritis patients have been reported from London, Newcastle, Epsom and Stevenage in the UK, as well as from Ireland, France, the Netherlands, Japan and Bermuda. *Proteus mirabilis* accounts for about 10% of all urinary tract infections (Fairley et al. 1971).

A. Ebringer, *Rheumatoid Arthritis and Proteus*,
DOI 10.1007/978-0-85729-950-5_11,
© Springer-Verlag London Limited 2012

However, the interesting observation was that no elevation was found in antibodies against the commonest microbe causing about 80% of urinary tract infections namely, *Escherichia coli*.

Thus, the elevation of antibodies only against *Proteus mirabilis* indicated that such immune responses were specific and could not be ascribed to nonspecific urinary tract infections occurring in patients whose manual dexterity had been compromised by arthritis or age.

If such had been the case, then an elevation in both anti-*Escherichia coli* antibodies and anti-*Proteus mirabilis* antibodies would have been expected, but only one of these microbes, namely *Proteus*, appeared to be involved in this arthritic disease.

Therefore, an investigation was carried out to determine whether the urine of patients with active rheumatoid arthritis contained *Proteus* bacteria.

The question was not whether there was overt bacterial infection in the urinary tract in the form of pyuria, as determined by finding 3,000 colony-forming units (CFU) per ml of urine, but whether there was an actual signal of the presence of *Proteus* bacteria, as measured by one colony-forming unit per ml of urine.

In 1993, Professor Israel Machtey from the Hasharon Hospital, Petach-Tiqva in Israel organised a meeting in Tel Aviv to discuss progress in rheumatology, and the results from our unit on urine cultures were published for the first time at this Symposium (Ebringer et al. 1993).

First Study with Rheumatoid Arthritis Patients, 'Disease Controls' and Healthy Controls

In the first study, mid-stream urine specimens were collected from 89 rheumatoid arthritis patients. There were 14 males and 75 females with a mean age of 43 years (range: 27–78 years) attending the Outpatient Clinics of the Department of Rheumatology at the Middlesex Hospital in London. The female to male ratio was 5.4:1.

The diagnosis of rheumatoid arthritis was made according to the criteria of the American Rheumatism Association (Ropes et al. 1958).

In addition to the use of non-steroidal anti-inflammatory drugs (NSAIDs), 50% of the rheumatoid arthritis patients were being treated with methotrexate and 20% with gold injections. Fewer than 10% of the rheumatoid arthritis patients were on steroids.

A further 37 non-rheumatoid arthritis patients with a diagnosis of osteoarthritis, psoriasis, ankylosing spondylitis, gout and systemic lupus erythematosus with a mean age of 45 years (range: 31–80 years) were also included in the study as 'disease controls'.

The specimens were coded in that only the surname and hospital number appeared on the label, and the microbiological tester did not know the sex, first name or the diagnosis of the patient providing the sample.

Since this method was designed to detect the presence or absence of microorganisms, with viable *Proteus* colonies being measured down to one colony-forming unit per ml of urine, it had to be calibrated against an age- and sex-matched healthy control population.

This proved to be quite a problem, but eventually two Church of England parishes were persuaded to provide mid-stream urine specimens over two Sundays.

A 'healthy parishioner' was defined as one who was attending church, hence mobile, had no history of arthritis and was not taking any drugs.

Once the project had been explained to the congregations, the response was enthusiastic and 234 samples were obtained from 115 men and 119 women, with ages ranging from 26 to 75 years.

Results of First Study

The mid-stream urine specimens were concentrated by centrifugation at 4,000 rpm for 20 min at 4°C. The pellet was suspended in 1 ml of nutrient broth (Oxoid), followed by inoculation onto cystine lactose electrolyte deficient agar (CLED;Oxoid) and plates incubated overnight aerobically at 37°C.

Suspect colonies were identified by standard microbiological methods and later confirmed using the API20E system (Bio Mérieux).

The frequency of isolation of *Proteus* microbes in the healthy controls was 11% (13/115) in men and 32% (38/119) in women.

The frequency of isolation of *Proteus* microbes in men with rheumatoid arthritis was 50% (7/14), and in women with rheumatoid arthritis, it was 63% (47/75) (Fig. 11.1).

Both of these observations were highly significant: when rheumatoid arthritis men were compared to healthy men (Chi square with Yates correction = 11.46, $p < 0.001$) and rheumatoid arthritis women with healthy women (Chi square with Yates correction = 16.43, $p < 0.001$).

The frequency of isolation of urinary *Proteus* in men with 'non-rheumatoid arthritis' was 7% (1/14), and in women with 'non-rheumatoid arthritis', it was 35% (8/23). These figures are similar to the ones obtained for healthy men (11%) and for healthy women (32%).

When the frequency of isolation of *Proteus* in rheumatoid arthritis women was compared to that in non-rheumatoid arthritis women, the difference was again statistically significant (Chi square with Yates correction = 4.48, $p < 0.05$), but the difference in isolation of *Proteus* bacteria between men with rheumatoid arthritis and men with 'non-rheumatoid arthritis' was not significant. However, the number of male patients in the 'non-rheumatoid arthritis' group was somewhat small.

This microbiological study has shown that rheumatoid arthritis patients attending an outpatient clinic have higher levels of viable urinary *Proteus* bacteria than comparable healthy controls of either sex or female 'disease controls' having non-rheumatoid arthritis.

Although the frequency of isolation of urinary *Proteus* in male rheumatoid arthritis patients was 50%, whilst it was only 7% in 'non-rheumatoid arthritis' patients, the number of

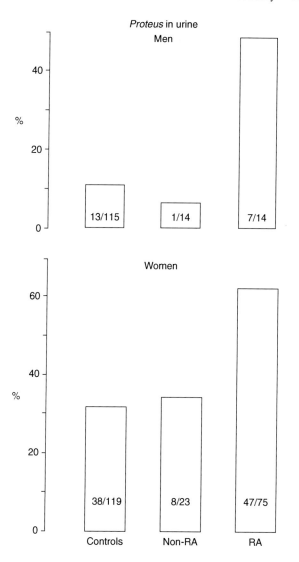

FIGURE 11.1 Percentage isolation of *Proteus* bacteria from the urines of rheumatoid arthritis patients, non-rheumatoid arthritis patients and healthy controls (From Ebringer et al. (1993))

patients in both groups was too small for this trend to be statistically significant.

Further studies are required to determine whether this trend in male rheumatoid arthritis patients compared to 'non-rheumatoid arthritis' patients will be confirmed by examining larger numbers of subjects.

However, this study has established that in over half of rheumatoid arthritis patients attending an Outpatient clinic, viable *Proteus* bacteria can be cultured from the urine when using sensitive methods of detection.

Thus, the source of the *Proteus* antigens, responsible for the specific elevation of anti-*Proteus* antibodies, would appear to be the *Proteus* bacteria located in the urinary tract.

This raises the question whether measures to treat urinary tract infections might have therapeutic relevance in the management of rheumatoid arthritis.

Second Study with Rheumatoid Arthritis Patients and Healthy Controls

In the second study, serum and urine samples were obtained from 20 rheumatoid arthritis patients, 5 were men and 15 were women. Their mean age was 58 years (range 33–81 years). The female to male ratio was 3/1.

Serum samples were also obtained from 20 healthy control subjects, 7 males and 13 females, and they had a mean age of 56 years (range: 35–80 years). None of the control subjects were taking any medication or had any arthritic symptoms.

The rheumatoid arthritis patients and control subjects in this second study were different from those investigated in the first study.

In the second study, mid-stream urine specimens were concentrated by centrifugation at 4,000 rpm for 20 min at 4°C, as previously described for the first study.

The pellet was resuspended in 1 ml of nutrient broth and tenfold dilutions made in glass tubes, followed by inoculation of a 25 μl aliquot onto CLED agar plates. The plates were incubated overnight aerobically at 37°C, suspect colonies identified and the results expressed as log number of colony-forming units (cfu) per millilitre of urine.

Enzyme-Linked Immunosorbent Assay

Enzyme-linked immunosorbent assays (ELISA) were carried as previously described.

Proteus mirabilis microbe was obtained from the urine sample of a rheumatoid arthritis patient, grown aerobically in nutrient broth, harvested and suspended in 0.15 M phosphate buffered saline (PBS pH 7.4). The stock solution was prepared to give an optical density (OD) at 540 nm of 0.25 on the spectrophotometer (Corning model 258) which is equivalent to 6×10^8 cells/ml.

The *Escherichia coli* microorganisms were obtained from the Department of Microbiology at King's College.

Mean OD units of IgG immunoglobulin antibody against *Proteus mirabilis* and *Escherichia coli* in the different groups were compared with Student's t-test, and the frequency of isolation of *Proteus mirabilis* was analysed by the Chi square statistic with Yates' correction.

Results of the Second Study

In the second study, the mean ($\pm$ standard error) level of IgG antibodies to *Proteus mirabilis* was 0.725 ± 0.096 OD units in rheumatoid arthritis patients and this was significantly higher than the mean level of 0.338 ± 0.055 OD units found in the healthy controls ($t = 5.46, p < 0.001$).

There was no significant elevation in IgG antibodies against *Escherichia coli* in rheumatoid arthritis patients when compared to controls (Fig. 11.2).

There was a positive correlation between anti-*Proteus* IgG antibody levels and the number of colony-forming units in

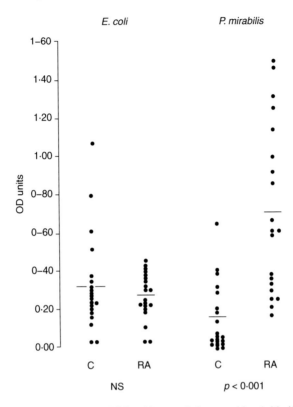

FIGURE 11.2 IgG in control (*C*) subjects and rheumatoid arthritis (*RA*) patients, when tested by ELISA against *Escherichia coli* and *Proteus mirabilis*. Bars=means (With kind permission from Wilson et al. (1997))

the 20 rheumatoid arthritis patients investigated ($r = +0.714$, $p < 0.001$) (Fig. 11.3).

Discussion and Conclusions

This microbiological study using sensitive culture methods shows that rheumatoid arthritis patients have higher levels of urinary *Proteus* than comparable healthy controls or patients having other arthritic diseases.

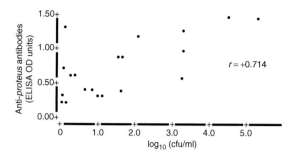

FIGURE 11.3 Correlation of anti-*Proteus* antibodies with *Proteus* colony-forming units: $\log_{10}$ cfu/ml (With kind permission from Wilson et al. (1997))

The frequency of isolation of *Proteus* in men with rheumatoid arthritis was 50%, and in women with rheumatoid arthritis it was even higher (Wilson et al. 1997).

Furthermore, antibody levels against *Proteus mirabilis* but not against *Escherichia coli* were elevated in these rheumatoid arthritis patients, thereby confirming previous studies from other geographical areas.

There was also a good correlation between anti-*Proteus* IgG antibodies found in serum and the number of urinary *Proteus* bacteria as measured by the number of colony-forming units per ml of urine.

These findings suggest that rheumatoid arthritis patients suffer from a subclinical and probably asymptomatic urinary infection by *Proteus mirabilis* but not by *Escherichia coli* bacteria. Similar results in rheumatoid arthritis patients have been reported from Dundee in Scotland (Senior et al. 1999).

However, a study from Newcastle could not find a significant difference in isolation rates of *Proteus mirabilis* in rheumatoid arthritis patients when compared to healthy controls (McDonagh et al. 1994).

These findings could be due to differences in methodology. In our study, we used a concentrated aliquot of urine, in an endeavour to detect subclinical infection, whilst McDonagh's group used non-concentrated urine for microbial detection.

These observations are relevant to the problem of the higher frequency of rheumatoid arthritis occurring in women since they also have a higher incidence of urinary tract infections.

The therapeutic implications of these results are quite clear. If *Proteus* microorganisms in the urinary tract are responsible for the elevation of anti-*Proteus* antibodies found in rheumatoid arthritis patients, then antibiotic and other measures could be undertaken, especially in early cases to prevent or delay the undesirable and crippling consequences so frequently encountered in this disease.

References

Ebringer A, Wilson C, Ahmadi K, Corbett M, Rashid T, Shipley M. Rheumatoid arthritis as a reactive arthritis to *Proteus* Infection: prospects for therapy. In: Machtey I, editor. Progress in rheumatology, vol. 5. Petach-Tiqva: Rheumatology Service, Hasharon Hospital; 1993. p. 77–83.

Fairley KF, Grounds AD, Carson NE, Laird EC, Gutch RC, McCallum PHG, et al. Site of infection in acute urinary tract infection in general practice. Lancet. 1971;2:615–8.

McDonagh J, Gray J, Sykes H, Walker DJ, Bint AS, Deighton CM. Anti-*Proteus* antibodies and *Proteus* organisms in rheumatoid arthritis: a clinical study. Br J Rheumatol. 1994;33:32–5.

Ropes MW, Bennet GA, Cobb S, Jacox R, Jessar RA. Revision of diagnostic criteria for rheumatoid arthritis. Bull Rheum Dis. 1958;9:175–6.

Senior BW, Anderson GA, Morley KD, Kerr MA. Evidence that patients with rheumatoid arthritis have asymptomatic 'non-significant' Proteus mirabilis bacteriuria more frequently than healthy controls. J Hyg. 1999;38:99–106.

Wilson C, Thakore A, Isenberg D, Ebringer A. Correlation between anti-*Proteus* antibodies and isolation rates of *Proteus mirabilis* in rheumatoid arthritis. Rheumatol Int. 1997;16:187–9.

Chapter 12
Molecular Similarity Between the 'Shared Epitope' of Rheumatoid Arthritis and Bacteria

Contents

Introduction: The Association of the 'Shared Epitope' EQR(K)RAA with Rheumatoid Arthritis

The association between rheumatoid arthritis and some subtypes of HLA-DR4 is well established not only in white subjects but also in many other ethnic groups. HLA-DR4 can be subdivided into several subtypes, only some of which are associated with rheumatoid arthritis (Stastny 1978).

In white subjects, DR4/Dw4 and DR4/Dw14 subtypes are associated with rheumatoid arthritis, whereas in Japanese subjects, it is DR4/Dw15 that is the susceptibility factor (Maeda et al. 1981).

A. Ebringer, *Rheumatoid Arthritis and Proteus*,
DOI 10.1007/978-0-85729-950-5_12,
© Springer-Verlag London Limited 2012

In Israel where DR4/Dw10 predominates, an association with HLA-DR1 has been reported in patients with rheumatoid arthritis (Schiff et al. 1982).

Analysis with synthetic oligonucleotides has shown that a particular region of the DRβ1 chain, from positions 70–74 coding for amino acids Gln-Arg-Arg-Ala-Ala (QRRAA), specific for DR1, Dw14 and Dw15, showed a strong association with rheumatoid arthritis compared to control subjects (Watanabe et al. 1989).

The sequence closely resembles that found in DRB1*0401 (DR4/Dw4) individuals, there being only one conservative substitution at position 71, from arginine to lysine (QKRAA). These two amino acids are positively charged, and thus the overall shape and charge configuration of these two sequences are similar.

This sequence EQ(K)RRAA has been described as the 'shared epitope' by the Winchester group from New York (Gregersen et al. 1987).

The glutamic acid (E) occupying position 69 is common to all DRβ1 molecules.

Furthermore, the EQRRAA sequence is also found in DRB1*1402 (DR6/DW16)-positive Yakima Indians affected by rheumatoid arthritis.

In contrast, the Dw10 haplotype has an aspartic acid at position 70 and glutamic acid at position 71, giving a net negative charge to the sequence, whereas Dw 13 has a glutamic acid at position 74.

The question arises as to whether there is 'molecular mimicry' between the EQR(K)RAA sequence and biological molecules found in the environment of rheumatoid arthritis patients.

Computer Analysis of the 'Shared Epitope' EQRRAA Sequence and the ESRRAL Sequence Found in the Haemolysins of *Proteus/Serratia* Microbes

The rheumatoid arthritis susceptibility sequence spanning residues 69–74 (EQRRAA) was used to scan published sequences of molecules from *Proteus* microorganisms. No

TABLE 12.1 Comparison of the charge distribution (+ positive, – negative; *N* neutral) of the amino acid sequences of HLA-DR1 and DR4 molecules with the similarity sequence in *Proteus mirabilis* membrane haemolysin

Disease link	Amino acid positions						HLA subtype
	69	70	71	72	73	74	
Associated with RA	–	N	+	+	N	N	DR1, Dw14, Dw15
	–	N	+	+	N	N	Dw4
	–	N	+	+	N	N	*Proteus* haemolysin
Not associated with RA	–	–	–	+	N	N	Dw10
	–	N	+	+	N	–	Dw13

RA rheumatoid arthritis

hexamer identity could be found in the Genbank database, but a closely related sequence (ESRRAL) spanning residues 32–37 of the surface membrane haemolysin of *Proteus mirabilis* (Hpm B polypeptide) was identified which had biochemical and charge similarity to the susceptibility sequence (Table 12.1).

A similar sequence was found in the membrane haemolysin of *Serratia marcescens* (Shl B polypeptide) but not in the haemolysins produced by ten other bacteria including *Escherichia coli* (Uphoff and Welch 1990).

The haemolysin molecule of *Proteus mirabilis* is composed of two polypeptides, Hpm B and Hpm A, with molecular weights of 63 and 165 kDa respectively. The Hpm B polypeptide is necessary for the extracellular secretion and activation of the structural haemolysin Hpm A and is thought to be located in the outer membrane where it could be involved in immune interactions. The ESRRAL sequence is hydrophilic and is an alpha helix (Fig. 12.1).

The secondary structure predictions were performed according to the published biochemical methods (Chou and Fasman 1978; Garnier et al. 1978).

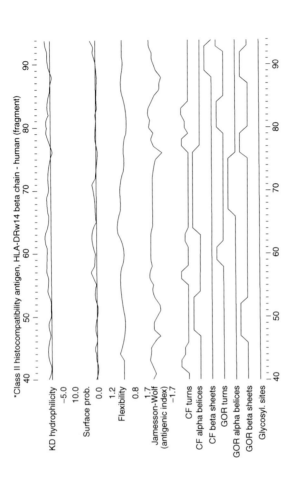

FIGURE 12.1 Computer plots generated from the amino acid sequences of **HLA-DRw14 β chain** and *Proteus haemolysin*. The hatched lines above and below the plots refer to the amino acid numbers of the protein sequence. Secondary structure predictions were performed according to published methods (Chou and Fasman 1978; Garnier et al. 1978)

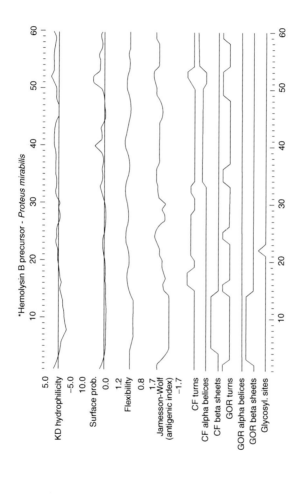

FIGURE 12.1 (continued)

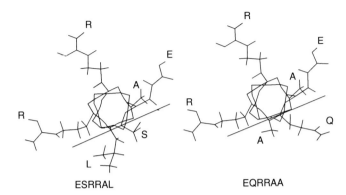

ESRRAL   EQRRAA

FIGURE 12.2 Helical models of ESRRAL and EQRRAA sequences. The predicted structures show a common charged surface of homologous residues available for immune interaction (*above line*). Modelling by DTMM (version 1.2) (Reprinted with permission from Springer Science+Business Media, Ebringer et al. (1992))

Molecular modelling of EQRRAA and ESRRAL motifs illustrates that the two sequences can be fitted to similar configurations producing almost identical antigenic epitopes (Fig. 12.2).

Implications for the Aetiology of Rheumatoid Arthritis

The similarity sequence of *Proteus mirabilis* membrane hae-molysin has the same charged amino acids arranged in the same order as the susceptibility sequence of DR1, Dw14 and Dw15 alleles, that is glutamic acid followed by a small neutral amino acid (serine) and then two positively charged arginines.

The three charged amino acids of the *Proteus mirabilis* sequence may provide an immunogenic group with a hydro-philicity value of +7.0, thereby indicating that it could be involved in immune interactions (Hopp and Woods 1981).

The important question is whether the *Proteus* peptide does indeed take up the predicted structure. If an antibody were to be produced against the similarity sequence of the *Proteus* haemolysin membrane protein, it may bind more readily to the DR1, Dw14 and Dw15 sequences, in addition to the Dw4, but not to the Dw10 and Dw13, as there are significant charge differences between these sequences.

Thus, the *Proteus* haemolysin sequence discriminates between alleles of HLA-DR1 and HLA-DR4 that are and are not associated with rheumatoid arthritis.

If such antibodies activate the complement cascade and stimulate natural killer cells, then this could provide an explanation for the association of the 'shared epitope' with rheumatoid arthritis.

Discussion and Conclusion

Computer analysis of the 'shared epitope' (EQRRAA) has identified a similarity sequence (ESRRAL) in both *Proteus* and *Serratia* microorganisms.

The question arises whether antibodies to these bacteria are relevant in the aetiology and pathogenesis of rheumatoid arthritis.

The results obtained by the Immunology group at King's College indicate that there is an amino acid homology between an outer membrane haemolysin protein of *Proteus haemolysin*, and *Serratia marcescens*, and the susceptibility sequence in HLA-DR1 and DR4 subtypes associated with rheumatoid arthritis (Ebringer et al. 1992).

References

Chou PY, Fasman G. Prediction of the secondary structure of proteins from the amino acid sequence. Adv Enzymol. 1978;47: 145–7.

Ebringer A, Cunningham P, Ahmadi K, Wrigglesworth J, Hosseini R, Wilson C. Sequence similarity between HLA-DR1 and DR4 subtypes associated with rheumatoid arthritis and *Proteus/Serratia* haemolysins. Ann Rheum Dis. 1992;51:1245–6.

Garnier J, Osguthorpe DJ, Robson BI. Analysis of the accuracy and implication of simple methods for predicting the secondary structure of globular proteins. J Mol Biol. 1978;120:97–120.

Gregersen PK, Silver J, Winchester RJ. The shared epitope hypothesis: an approach to understanding the molecular genetics of susceptibility to rheumatoid arthritis. Arthritis Rheum. 1987;30:1205–13.

Hopp TP, Woods KR. Prediction of protein antigenic determinants from amino acid sequences. Proc Natl Acad Sci USA. 1981;78: 3824–8.

Maeda H, Juji T, Mitsui H, Sonozaki H, Okitsu H. HLA-DR4 and rheumatoid arthritis in Japanese people. Ann Rheum Dis. 1981;40:299–302.

Schiff B, Mizrachi Y, Orgad S, Yaron M, Gazit E. Association of HLA-Aw31 and HLA-DR1 with adult rheumatoid arthritis. Ann Rheum Dis. 1982;41:403–4.

Stastny P. Association of the B-cell alloantigen DRW4 with rheumatoid arthritis. N Engl J Med. 1978;298:869–71.

Uphoff TS, Welch RA. Nucleotide sequencing of the *Proteus mirabilis* calcium independent haemolysin genes (hpm A and hpm B) reveals sequence similarity with the *Serratia marcescens* haemolysin genes (shl A and shl B). J Bacteriol. 1990;170:3177–88.

Watanabe Y, Tokunaga K, Matsuki K, Takeuchi F, Matsuta K, Maeda A, et al. Putative amino acid sequence of HLA DRβ chain contributing to rheumatoid arthritis susceptibility. J Exp Med. 1989;169:2263–8.

Chapter 13
The 'Shared Epitope', *Proteus* Haemolysin, Type XI Collagen and Rheumatoid Arthritis

Contents

A. Ebringer, *Rheumatoid Arthritis and Proteus*,
DOI 10.1007/978-0-85729-950-5_13,
© Springer-Verlag London Limited 2012

Introduction: The Association of the 'Shared Epitope' EQ(K)RRAA with the ESRRAL Sequence of *Proteus* Haemolysin and the Link of *Proteus* Urease with Collagen

The association between rheumatoid arthritis and some sub-types of HLA-DR4 is well known and a particular region of the DRβ1 chain, from positions 70–74 coding for amino acids Gln-Arg-Arg-Ala-Ala (QRRAA) and found in DRB1*0101 (DR1) and some DR4 subtypes DRB1*0404 (DW14) and DRB1*0405 (Dw15), has been identified as the molecular sequence responsible for the susceptibility to rheumatoid arthritis (Nepom et al. 1989).

This susceptibility sequence has been given the name of the 'shared epitope'.

The sequence closely resembles that found in DRB1*0401 (DR4/Dw4) individuals, there being only one conservative substitution at position 71, from arginine to lysine (QKRAA). These two amino acids are positively charged, and thus the overall shape and charge configuration of these two sequences are similar.

The glutamic acid occupying position 69 is common to all DRβ1 molecules.

Our group has reported an amino acid homology between an outer membrane haemolysin protein of *Proteus mirabilis* and the 'shared epitope' found in patients with rheumatoid arthritis.

Early studies from our laboratory showed that anti-HLA-DR4 tissue typing sera bound significantly to *Proteus mirabilis* compared to non-HLA-DR4 tissue typing sera, but no such interaction was found with *Escherichia coli* bacteria.

The hexamer sequence ESRRAL of *Proteus mirabilis* hae-molysin is hydrophilic which suggests that it may be immuno-genic and could be involved in antibody interactions.

The present study was undertaken to compare the spatial configurations of EQRRAA/ESRRAL sequences for similarity using molecular modelling, and to determine if antibodies to the

ESRRAL peptide and to other similarity sequences of *Proteus mirabilis* were present in active rheumatoid arthritis patients.

Investigations were also carried out to determine if there was any link between *Proteus* bacteria and collagens.

Molecular Modelling of ESRRAL from *Proteus* with EQRRAA of HLA-DR1/4

Comparison of space filling models of a predicted ESRRAL sequence of *Proteus* haemolysin and EQRRAA sequence within DRB1*0101 (HLA-DR1) from known crystallographic structure was carried out to study spatial configuration. The ESRRAL model was constructed as a helix with torsional angles corresponding to those observed in the known EQRRAA sequence and the two sequences were superimposed (root mean square (RMS) = 0.046).

The ESRRAL and EQRRAA sequences were also compared with the sequence EDERAA present in DRB1*0402 (HLA-DR4/Dw10) which is not associated with rheumatoid arthritis.

Molecular modelling of the two structures ESRRAL and EQRRAA showed a common surface of homologous residues. The positions 32, 34, 35 and 69, 71, 72 form a motif common to HLA-DR and *Proteus mirabilis* occupying the same stereochemical space.

However, the EDERAA sequence of DRB1*0402 (HLA-DR4/Dw10), which is not associated with rheumatoid arthritis, differed from both the ESRRAL and EQRRAA motifs (Fig. 13.1).

Molecular Modelling of IRRET from *Proteus* Urease with LRREI of Type XI Hyaline Cartilage

Rheumatoid arthritis is a systemic disorder and cartilage destruction is a major feature of the disease. Therefore, a search of the protein database was made for any sequence of

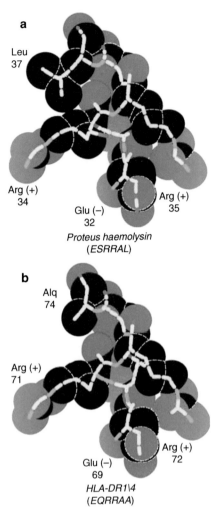

a

Leu
37

Arg (+)
34

Glu (–)
32

Arg (+)
35

Proteus haemolysin
(ESRRAL)

b

Alq
74

Arg (+)
71

Glu (–)
69

Arg (+)
72

HLA-DR1\4
(EQRRAA)

FIGURE 13.1 Comparison of space filling models. (**a**) ESRRAL sequence of *Proteus mirabilis* haemolysin predicted from known crystallographic structure. (**b**) EQRRAA sequence within DRB1*0101 (HLA-DR1), predicted from known crystallographic structure. (**c**) EDERAA sequence of DRB1*0402 (HLA-DR4/Dw10), an HLA group not associated with rheumatoid arthritis (Reprinted with permission from Springer Science+Business Media, Wilson et al. (1995))

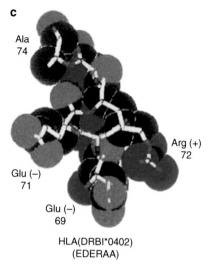

c

Ala
74

Arg (+)
72

Glu (−)
71

Glu (−)
69

HLA(DRBI*0402)
(EDERAA)

FIGURE 13.1 (continued)

Proteus mirabilis showing some 'molecular mimicry' or structural similarity to any collagens.

One way of distinguishing urine cultures is by determining whether the bacterial colonies obtained are either urease-positive or urease-negative. Urease is not present in *Escherichia coli* but is present in *Proteus* bacteria. Thus, the hypothetical question arose if the *Proteus* urease molecule had any similarity or showed any 'molecular mimicry' to collagens known to be present in joint tissues, hyaline cartilage and tendons.

A computer analysis was carried out to determine if there was any molecular association between *Proteus* urease and collagens.

An amino acid homology was identified between *Proteus mirabilis* urease (IRRET), amino acid residues 421–425 and α2(XI) collagen (LRREI) residues 421–425 (Kimura et al. 1989).

Type XI collagen is a component of hyaline cartilage which is composed of three different polypeptide subunits α1(XI), α2(XI) and α3(XI).

Northern blot analysis shows that the α2(XI) collagen gene is expressed in hyaline cartilage but not in adult liver, skin or tendons.

Comparison of space filling models was made of the predicted IRRET sequence of *Proteus mirabilis* urease and LRREI of α2(XI) collagen. Both sequences were constructed as helices and the two sequences superimposed (RMS = 0.011). Structures were modelled using Alchemy III (Tripos ASSOC Inc, St. Louis, USA).

Molecular modelling of the two sequences IRRET and LRREI also showed a common surface of homologous residues.

The positions 338, 339, 340 and 421, 422, 423 form a motif common to type XI collagen and *Proteus mirabilis* urease occupying the same stereochemical space (Fig. 13.2).

The common surface of homologous residues observed in the sequences ESRRAL/EQRRAA and IRRET/LRREI, which may be involved in immune interactions, consists of two positively charged arginines and one negatively charged glutamic acid.

First Study with Rheumatoid Arthritis Patients, Measuring Antibodies Against ESRRAL and the *Proteus* Haemolysin Protein

Sera were collected from active rheumatoid arthritis patients having an erythrocyte sedimentation rate above 15 mm/h. The rheumatoid arthritis patients were attending the Rheumatology Department at the Lister Hospital in Stevenage, Herts and active ankylosing spondylitis patients, who acted as 'disease controls' were attending the 'Ankylosing Spondylitis Research Clinic' of the Middlesex Hospital.

The diagnosis of rheumatoid arthritis was made according to the American Rheumatism Association criteria, and the diagnosis of ankylosing spondylitis was made according to the New York criteria.

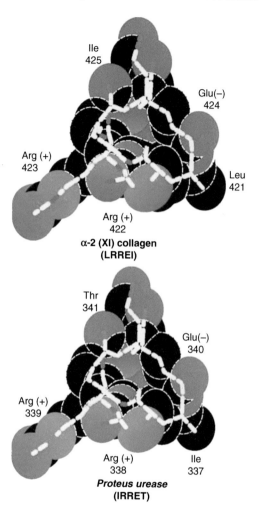

FIGURE 13.2 Space filling model of **LRREI** sequence of α2(XI) collagen, predicted from known crystallographic structure and **IRRET** sequence of *Proteus mirabilis* urease predicted from known crystallographic structure (Reprinted with permission from Springer Science+Business Media, Wilson et al. (1995))

In the first study, antibodies were measured against the ESRRAL peptide and the *Proteus* haemolysin protein.

Sera were obtained from 40 rheumatoid arthritis. Their mean age was 59 years (range: 37–77 years), and there were 10 men and 30 women. Their mean erythrocyte sedimentation rate (± standard error) was 46.2 ± 4.0 mm/h. The female to male ratio in the rheumatoid arthritis patients was 3:1.

Sera were also obtained from 30 ankylosing spondylitis patients. Their mean age was 49 years (range: 27–76 years), and there were 23 men and 7 women. The male to female ratio was 3.3:1. Their mean erythrocyte sedimentation rate (± standard error) was 30.1 ± 5.2 mm/h.

There were also 30 healthy control subjects. Their mean age was 23 years (range: 21–27 years). There were 15 male and 15 female healthy control subjects.

ELISA Studies with (a) Synthetic Peptides and (b) *Proteus* Haemolysin Protein

Synthetic Peptides

Peptides were prepared by solid phase synthesis and analysed for purity by high-performance liquid chromatography as previously described.

The test peptide was LGSIS**ESRRAL**QDSQR (16-mer), which represents amino acid residues 27–42 of *Proteus mirabilis* haemolysin (hpm B) and has in its middle the ESRRAL sequence.

The control peptide SQKDIL**EDERAA**VDTY (16-mer) from DRB1*0402 (HLA-DR4/Dw10) was used for comparison. It has in its middle the EDERAA sequence and this HLA group is not associated with rheumatoid arthritis.

Two other control peptides, YASGASGAS (9-mer) and DAHKSEVAHRFLDLGEENFKALVL (24-mer), were used to exclude nonspecific binding.

Sera were tested against the *Proteus mirabilis* haemolysin peptide and control peptides by enzyme-linked immunosorbent assay (ELISA), as previously described.

All assays were carried out under code, so that the status of each serum sample under investigation was not known to the tester.

Antibodies to the *Proteus mirabilis* haemolysin peptide LGSIS**ESRRAL**QDSQR, of the IgG class, containing in the middle the ESRRAL sequence, were significantly elevated in rheumatoid arthritis patients when compared to ankylosing spondylitis patients or healthy controls. The mean (± standard error) in rheumatoid arthritis patients was 0.263 ± 0.011 OD units and this was significantly higher than the mean in ankylosing spondylitis patients which was 0.162 ± 0.012 OD units ($t = 5.98, p < 0.001$) or the mean in healthy control subjects which was 0.158 ± 0.014 OD units ($t = 5.90, p < 0.001$) (Fig. 13.3).

There was no significant reactivity by the rheumatoid arthritis patients or ankylosing spondylitis patients against the DRB1*0402 (HLA-DR4/Dw10) SQKDIL**EDERAA**VDTY (16-mer) peptide, an HLA group not associated with rheumatoid arthritis when compared to controls.

Proteus Haemolysin

Purification of the 63-kDa outer membrane haemolysin protein was carried as originally described for *Escherichia coli* (Schnaitman 1974).

Sera obtained from the same subjects as above were tested against *Proteus mirabilis* haemolysin (63 kDa) protein and against two control haemolysin proteins, obtained from *Streptococcus pyogenes* and *Vibrio parahaemolyticus* (Sigma Chemical Company Ltd) by ELISA.

Briefly, polystyrene microtitre plates (Dynatech) were coated with the haemolysin protein (2.0 µg/well) and incubated overnight at 4°C. Serum samples were diluted 1/200 in PBS-Tween and the plates saturated with 0.1% BSA-PBS-Tween. The remainder of the assay procedure was as previously described for the synthetic peptides.

The difference between the titres in ankylosing spondylitis patients and healthy controls, when tested against the *Proteus mirabilis* haemolysin, was not significant.

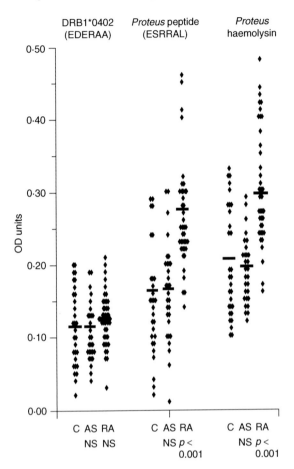

F<small>IGURE</small> 13.3 Antibody titres for IgG immunoglobulin in controls (*C*) and patients with ankylosing spondylitis (*AS*) or rheumatoid arthritis (*RA*) when tested by ELISA against the synthetic peptides EDERAA, ESRRAL and the haemolysin protein of *Proteus mirabilis*. *OD* optical density. Bars indicate means. *NS* not significant when compared to controls (Reprinted with permission from Springer Science+Business Media, Wilson et al. (1995))

There was no elevation in IgA and IgM antibodies against the *Proteus* haemolysin peptide.

However, antibodies of the IgG class to *Proteus mirabilis* haemolysin protein (63 kDa) were significantly elevated in rheumatoid arthritis patients when compared to ankylosing spondylitis patients and healthy controls.

The mean (± standard error) in rheumatoid arthritis patients was 0.304 ± 0.013 OD units and this was significantly higher than the mean in ankylosing spondylitis patients which was 0.190 ± 0.075 OD units ($t = 7.11, p < 0.001$) or the mean in healthy control subjects which was 0.201 ± 0.014 OD units ($t = 5.52, p < 0.001$) (Fig. 13.3).

In contrast, there was no elevation in IgA or IgM antibodies against the *Proteus* haemolysin protein and no significant reactivity by the rheumatoid arthritis patients against the two control *Streptococcus pyogenes* and *Vibrio parahaemolyticus* haemolysin proteins.

Second Study with Rheumatoid Arthritis Patients, Measuring Antibodies Against Urease Proteins

In the second study, antibodies were measured against two different preparations of bacterial urease, one from *Bacillus pasteurii* urease and the other one from *Proteus mirabilis* urease.

Sera were obtained from 20 rheumatoid arthritis patients. Their mean age was 56 years (range: 20–75 years), and there were 5 men and 15 women. The female to male ratio in the rheumatoid arthritis patients was 3:1. Their mean (± standard error) erythrocyte sedimentation rate was 59.8 ± 7.7 mm/h.

Sera were also obtained from 40 ankylosing spondylitis patients. Their mean age was 45 years (range: 21–76 years). There were 29 men and 11 women. The male to female ratio in the ankylosing spondylitis patients was 2.6:1. Their mean (± standard error) erythrocyte sedimentation rate was 25.9 ± 3.6 mm/h.

There were also 15 healthy control subjects and their mean age was 29 years (range: 21–52 years).

Purification of the 280-kDa *Proteus mirabilis* urease protein was carried out by the method of Jones and Mobley (Jones and Mobley 1989).

Sera were obtained from different subjects than the ones investigated in the first study and were tested against *Proteus mirabilis* urease protein and *Bacillus pasteurii* urease (Sigma Chemical Company) by ELISA. Polystyrene microtitre plates (Dynatech) were coated with the urease protein (2 μg/well) and assays carried out as before.

Antibody titres against *Proteus mirabilis* urease protein of the IgG class were significantly elevated in rheumatoid arthritis patients when compared to ankylosing spondylitis patients or healthy controls.

The mean (± standard error) in rheumatoid arthritis patients was 0.68 ± 0.07 OD units and this was significantly higher than the mean in ankylosing spondylitis patients which was 0.39 ± 0.02 OD units ($t = 5.09$, $p < 0.001$) or the mean in healthy control subjects which was 0.32 ± 0.04 OD units ($t = 4.06$, $p < .001$), but there was no significant difference in the titres between ankylosing spondylitis patients and healthy controls (Fig. 13.4).

Furthermore, there was no significant reactivity by rheumatoid arthritis patients against *Bacillus pasteurii* urease (Fig. 13.4).

Discussion and Conclusions

In this study, active patients with rheumatoid arthritis have been shown to have an increased titre of antibodies against a synthetic peptide derived from *Proteus mirabilis* membrane haemolysin (hpm B), containing the hexamer sequence ESRRAL which is homologous with the rheumatoid arthritis susceptibility sequence EQ(K)RRAA of the DRβ1 chain of class II major histocompatibility complex molecules.

Rheumatoid arthritis patients were also found to have an elevated titre of antibodies against the native *Proteus*

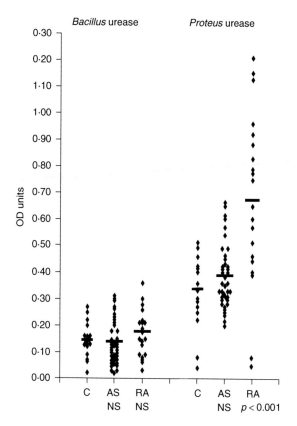

FIGURE 13.4 Antibody titres for IgG immunoglobulin in controls (*C*) and patients with ankylosing spondylitis (*AS*) or rheumatoid arthritis (*RA*) when tested by ELISA against the urease proteins of *Proteus mirabilis* and *Bacillus pasteurii*. *OD* optical density. Bars indicate means. *NS* not significant when compared to controls (Reprinted with permission from Springer Science+Business Media, Wilson et al. (1995))

haemolysin protein but not against the haemolysin proteins found in *Streptococcus pyogenes* or *Vibrio parahaemolyticus*.

The ESRRAL motif was found in three of 67,000 sequences: *Proteus mirabilis*, *Serratia marcescens* and *Vibrio cholerae*.

This demonstration of a significant increase in IgG but not IgA antibodies to *Proteus mirabilis* membrane haemolysin sequence and to the native protein suggests that the site of infection in rheumatoid arthritis patients is not a mucosal surface involving IgA but in some interstitial tissue leading to IgG production.

In a related study, autoantibodies against a 16-mer synthetic peptide of DRB1*0405 (HLA-DR4/Dw15) β1 chain, containing the EQRRAA sequence, were reported to be increased in Japanese patients with rheumatoid arthritis, when tested by ELISA (Takeuchi et al. 1990).

This study also shows that rheumatoid arthritis patients have an increased titre of antibodies to the urease protein derived from *Proteus mirabilis*, containing a sequence IRRET which is homologous with sequence LRREI present in type XI collagen. The IRRET sequence was found in six biological proteins: *Bacillus sphaericus*, murine leukaemia virus, *Escherichia coli*, *Klebsiella aerogenes*, *Proteus vulgaris* and *Proteus mirabilis* out of 30,000 sequences examined in the protein database. The high level of *Proteus mirabilis* antibodies was not attributable to nonspecific effects of inflammation because the ankylosing spondylitis patients also had increased erythrocyte sedimentation rates, yet their levels of *Proteus mirabilis* antibodies were similar to those found in healthy control subjects.

The ESRRAL and IRRET sequences are both hydrophilic and in helical configurations where they may be involved in immune interactions.

The results of this study suggest that rheumatoid arthritis patients have a significant increase in antibodies to a *Proteus* membrane haemolysin sequence containing a hexamer which is homologous with the rheumatoid arthritis susceptibility sequence described by the 'shared epitope'.

Moreover, the rheumatoid arthritis patients in this study also had a significant elevation in antibodies to *Proteus mirabilis* urease containing a pentamer which is homologous with a sequence in type XI collagen (Wilson et al. 1995).

Further investigations are required to determine if antibodies to ESRRAL/IRRET and haemolysin/urease react with HLA alleles and collagen to produce tissue damage, thereby contributing to the pathogenesis of this disease.

References

Jones BD, Mobley HLT. *Proteus mirabilis* urease: nucleotide sequence determination and comparison with jack bean urease. J Bacteriol. 1989;171:6414–22.

Kimura T, Cheah KSE, Chan SDH, Lui VC, Mattei MG, van der Rest M, et al. The human α2 collagen (COLIIA2) chain molecular cloning of cDNA and genomic DNA reveals characteristics of a fibrillar collagen with differences in genomic organisation. J Biol Chem. 1989;264:13910–6.

Nepom GT, Byers P, Seyfried CR. HLA genes associated with rheumatoid arthritis. Identification of susceptibility genes using oligonucleotide probes. Arthritis Rheum. 1989;33:15–21.

Schnaitman CA. Outer membrane proteins of Escherichia Coli 0 III. J Bacteriol. 1974;118:442–53.

Takeuchi F, Kosuge E, Matsuta K, Nakano K, Tokunaga K, Juji T, et al. Antibody to a specific HLA-DR β1 sequence in Japanese patients with rheumatoid arthritis. Arthritis Rheum. 1990;33:1867–8.

Wilson C, Ebringer A, Ahmadi K, Wrigglesworth J, Tiwana H, Fielder M, et al. Shared amino acid sequences between major histocompatibility complex class II glycoproteins, type XI collagen and *Proteus mirabilis* in rheumatoid arthritis. Ann Rheum Dis. 1995;54:216–20.

Chapter 14
Gram-Negative Bacteria Possess Sequences Which Resemble the 'Shared Epitope' but Only *Proteus* Infect Rheumatoid Arthritis Patients

Contents

A. Ebringer, *Rheumatoid Arthritis and Proteus*,
DOI 10.1007/978-0-85729-950-5_14,
© Springer-Verlag London Limited 2012

Introduction: The ESRRAL Sequence of *Proteus* Haemolysin Is Also Found in Three Other Gram-Negative Bacteria

The 'shared epitope' EQRRAA has been found to resemble or show 'molecular mimicry' with the sequence ESRRAL spanning residues 32–37 of the surface membrane haemolysin of *Proteus mirabilis* (Hpm B polypeptide).

The same hexamer sequence was also found in the membrane haemolysin of *Serratia marcescens* (Shl B polypeptide).

Furthermore, homologous sequences were also found in *Escherichia coli* (QKRAA) and in *Pseudomonas aeruginosa* (DQRRAA).

This study was undertaken to investigate whether active rheumatoid arthritis patients have antibodies to these other Gram-negative microorganisms.

Sera from Rheumatoid Arthritis Patients and Controls

Sera were obtained from active rheumatoid arthritis patients, having an erythrocyte sedimentation rate greater than 15 mm/h and attending the Rheumatology Department at the Lister Hospital in Stevenage. Sera were also obtained from active anky-losing spondylitis patients attending the 'Ankylosing Spondylitis Research Clinic' of the Middlesex Hospital. The diagnosis of rheumatoid arthritis was according to the American Rheumatism Association criteria and that of ankylosing spondylitis by the New York criteria. Sera from healthy control subjects were sup-plied by the Blood Transfusion Service in London.

In the study, total immunoglobulin antibodies were mea-sured in 181 individuals against *Serratia marcescens*, *Proteus mirabilis*, *Escherichia coli* and *Pseudomonas aeruginosa*.

The groups examined were as follows: 60 patients with rheumatoid arthritis (21 male; 45 female) with a mean age of

48 years (range: 20–71 years) and having a mean (± standard error) erythrocyte sedimentation rate 43.4±4.3 mm/h. The female to male ratio was 2.1:1.

There were also 61 ankylosing spondylitis patients (49 male; 12 female) with a mean age of 46 years (range: 24–73 years) and having a mean (± standard error) erythrocyte sedimentation rate 42.9±9.5 mm/h and 60 healthy control subjects (30 male; 30 female) with a mean age of 34 years (range: 19–66 years).

Enzyme Immunosorbent Assay (ELISA)

Serratia marcescens, *Proteus mirabilis*, *Escherichia coli* and *Pseudomonas aeruginosa* were clinical isolates obtained from the Department of Microbiology at King's College, London. Cultures were prepared and ELISA carried out, as previously described.

The C-reactive protein levels were determined by the single radial immunodiffusion method of Mancini and the results expressed as mg/L of serum.

Antibody Results Against the Four Gram-Negative Bacteria

Antibodies to *Proteus mirabilis* of total (IgA + IgG + IgM) immunoglobulin were significantly elevated in the active rheumatoid arthritis patients compared to active ankylosing spondylitis patients or healthy controls. The mean ± (standard error) in rheumatoid arthritis patients was 0.869±0.054 OD units and this was significantly higher than the mean in active ankylosing spondylitis patients which was 0.228±0.012 ($t=11.30$, $p<0.001$) or the mean in healthy control subjects which was 0.214±0.015 ($t=11.22$, $p<0.001$) (Fig. 14.1).

There was no significant difference in antibody levels between the active ankylosing spondylitis patients and healthy controls.

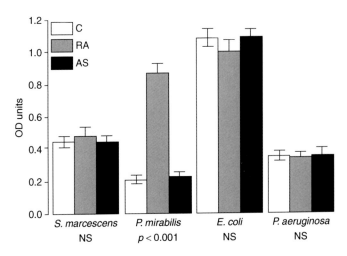

FIGURE 14.1 Total immunoglobulin titres (mean ± standard error) in *Serratia marcescens*, *Proteus mirabilis*, *Escherichia coli* and *Pseudomonas aeruginosa* in 60 healthy controls (*C*), 60 active rheumatoid arthritis (*RA*) and 61 active ankylosing spondylitis (*AS*) patients. (*N.S.* not significant) (Reprinted with kind permission from Tiwana et al. (1996))

There was no significant reactivity in the rheumatoid arthritis or ankylosing spondylitis patients against *Pseudomonas aeruginosa*, *Serratia marcescens* or *Escherichia coli* when compared to the healthy controls (Fig. 14.1).

The reproducibility of the assay for each sample was tested by calculating the coefficient of variation. The coefficients of variation for *Serratia marcescens*, *Proteus mirabilis*, *Escherichia coli* and *Pseudomonas aeruginosa* were calculated to be 4%, 5%, 7% and 4% respectively.

The mean ± (standard error) C-reactive protein level was significantly higher in both the rheumatoid arthritis patients 40.4 ± 9.4 mg/l ($t = 7.29$, $p < 0.001$)(range: 0–160) and ankylosing spondylitis patients 34.0 ± 3.3 mg/l ($t = 5.85$, $p < 0.001$) (range: 0–108) when compared to the mean in controls which was 12.0 ± 1.6 mg/l (range:1–37).

Discussion and Conclusions

In this study, active patients with rheumatoid arthritis have been shown to have an increased levels of total immuno-globulin (IgA + IgG + IgM) against whole *Proteus mirabilis* microorganisms but no elevations against the three other Gram-negative bacteria namely *Serratia marcescens*, *Escherichia coli* and *Pseudomonas aeruginosa* which are known to carry ESRRAL or a homologous sequence.

It has been reported that rheumatoid arthritis patients with early disease exhibit high antibody titres to a 15-mer synthetic peptide of the dnaJ heat shock protein of *Escherichia coli* (Albani et al. 1995) This heat shock protein also contains the EQKRAA sequence found in the susceptibility sequences of HLA molecules associated with rheumatoid arthritis.

The susceptibility sequence EQKRAA is also found in the dnaJ heat shock protein of Epstein–Barr virus and a mimicking sequence DQRRAA is also found in the isoamy-lase precursor of *Pseudomonas aeruginosa* with a conservative substitution of glutamic acid (E) for aspartic acid (D) (Table 14.1).

However, there does not appear to be any antibody elevations in rheumatoid arthritis patients against either *Escherichia coli* or *Pseudomonas aeruginosa*.

The ESRRAL sequence is also present in *Vibrio cholerae* and *Brucella ovis* (Protein Information data base (PIR) release 44). However, these microorganisms are highly pathogenic and therefore unlikely to persist in patients following recovery. It is unlikely that they play a role in the onset of a chronic disease.

For a chronic autoimmune disease, one requires a mildly pathogenic microbe, causing almost an asymptomatic disease with a continuous and florid production of antibodies which bind to cross-reactive self-antigens and when present in high titres will activate the complement cascade and NK cells which then lead to tissue damage at a site distal from the original site of infection. Such anti-bacterial antibodies binding to self-tissues will then be known as autoantibodies.

TABLE 14.1 Comparison of amino acid sequences of HLA-DRβ1 chain, spanning residues 69–74 and microorganisms retrieved from PIR release 44 which have similar sequences in other proteins

Source	Amino acids	Positions	Location
DRβ1 chain	EQRRAA	69–74	DR1, DR4/Dw14, Dw15, DR6/Dw16
Epstein–Barr virus	EQRRAA	807–812	dnaJ heat shock protein
E. coli	EQRRAA	61–65	dnaJ heat shock protein
P. aeruginosa	DQRRAA	579–584	dnaJ heat shock protein
P. mirabilis	ESRRAL	32–37	Haemolysin B precursor
S. marcescens	ESRRAL	34–39	Haemolysin (Shl B)
V. cholerae	ESRRAL	19–24	Methyltransferase-adenine specific precursor
B. ovis	ESRRAL	107–112	Isoamylase precursor

PIR Protein Information Resource data base

This model occurs in rheumatic fever, and it is not inconceivable that a similar process might occur with rheumatoid arthritis patients when they produce high titres of anti-*Proteus* antibodies.

Further evidence for a role of microorganisms in the aetiology of rheumatoid arthritis is illustrated by the use of antimicrobial agents such as minocycline which have been shown to reduce joint tenderness and swelling and also a decrease in inflammatory parameters such as C-reactive protein and erythrocyte sedimentation rates (Langewitz et al. 1992).

In a double-blind placebo-controlled trial, a group from the Netherlands have shown that minocycline is effective in some patients with rheumatoid arthritis (Kloppenburg et al. 1994).

Finally one must mention Professor Thomas McPherson Brown (1906–1989) who graduated from the John Hopkins Medical School in Baltimore (Maryland) and spent his lifetime investigating rheumatoid arthritis. Whilst at the Rockefeller Institute in New York, he developed the concept that antibiotic therapy, especially minocycline, might be beneficial in the treatment of rheumatoid arthritis. His results have been confirmed by many centres, the question arises, which bacteria were involved, mycoplasma or the *Proteus* bacteria as suggested by these studies. Both mycoplasmas and *Proteus* bacteria respond to minocycline therapy, and clearly further investigations are required to resolve these questions.

References

Albani S, Keystone EC, Nelson L. Positive selection in autoimmunity: abnormal immune responses to a bacterial dnaJ antigenic determinant in patients with early rheumatoid arthritis. Nat Med. 1995;1:448–52.

Kloppenburg M, Breedveld FC, Terwiel J, Mallee C, Dijkmans RAC. Minocycline in active rheumatoid arthritis: a double blind, placebo controlled trial. Arthritis Rheum. 1994;37:629–36.

Langewitz P, Bank I, Zemer D, Book M. Treatment of resistant rheumatoid arthritis with minocycline: an open study. J Rheumatol. 1992;19:1502–4.

Tiwana H, Wilson C, Cunningham P, Binder A, Ebringer A. Antibodies to four gram-negative bacteria in Rheumatoid Arthritis which share sequences with the Rheumatoid Arthritis susceptibility motif. Oxford University Press, Br J Rheumatol. 1996;35:592–594.

Chapter 15
Immune Responses to *Proteus* in Rheumatoid Arthritis Patients from Finland and Japan

Contents

A. Ebringer, *Rheumatoid Arthritis and Proteus*,
DOI 10.1007/978-0-85729-950-5_15,
© Springer-Verlag London Limited 2012

Finland and Japan: Introduction

In 2003, Dr. Marjatta Leirisalo and Dr. Leena Paimela from Helsinki brought sera from rheumatoid arthritis patients to London to be investigated for antibodies to *Proteus* as well as against peptide sequences crossreacting with HLA-DR1/4 antigens.

Dr. Kobayashi from the Juntendo University in Tokyo indicated also his interest to participate in this study.

A total of 230 serum samples obtained from Finnish patients and two Japanese centres in Tokyo and Otsu, with patients having either rheumatoid arthritis or systemic lupus erythematosus and blood donors, were available for study. The study was carried out under coded conditions in the Immunology Unit at King's College in London.

Antibodies to *Proteus* peptides had only been carried out previously in English rheumatoid arthritis patients but not in rheumatoid arthritis patients originating from other countries.

The aim was to establish whether specific antibodies to *Proteus* and to *Proteus* sequences could be demonstrated in rheumatoid arthritis patients from other countries such as Finland and Japan.

Helsinki: Location and History

Helsinki is the capital of Finland and has a population of over half a million. Finland was under Swedish sovereignty for over six centuries from 1150 to 1809.

Helsinki was founded in 1550 by the Swedish king Gustav Vasa. When the Grand Duchy of Finland came under Russian control in 1809, the capital of Finland was transferred from Turku to Helsinki.

During the nineteenth century, the use of the Finnish language increased in Helsinki as there was a migration from the countryside to towns. However, Finland has still two official languages, Finnish and Swedish.

In 1917, Finland declared its independence from Russia and Helsinki became a prosperous town and the cultural centre of the country.

During the Second World War, Finland courageously defended its independence from the Soviet Union.

Finnish medicine is renowned for its scientific accuracy, originality and extensive epidemiological studies which cover and involve the whole nation.

Tokyo: Location and History

Tokyo also known as the 'Eastern Capital' is located in the south-eastern side of the main island of Honshu. Tokyo was originally a small fishing village named Edo.

In 1590, the shogun Tokugawa Ieyasu made Edo his capital. During the Edo period, Tokyo grew into one of the largest cities in the world.

In 1869, the Emperor Meiji moved the capital from Kyoto to Tokyo.

Tokyo has now a population of over eight million but the Greater Area of Tokyo is a huge conurbation or metropolis of 35 million people.

Juntendo University of Tokyo was established in 1838 and is the oldest school of Western medicine in Japan.

Patients and Controls

A total of 230 serum samples obtained from patients with rheumatoid arthritis and systemic lupus erythematosus as well as healthy subjects were collected in Finland and Japan.

They were investigated for anti-bacterial and anti-peptide antibody levels using indirect immunofluorescence and enzyme-linked immunosorbent assay (ELISA).

Among these sera, 129 coded samples were obtained from a Finnish population consisting of 72 patients with 'Early rheumatoid arthritis' and 27 patients with 'Advanced rheumatoid arthritis' attending the Second Department of Medicine of the University of Helsinki.

'Early Rheumatoid Arthritis' was defined as a disease that was present for less than 12 months and 'Advanced Rheumatoid Arthritis' was a disease present in a patient for more than 12 months.

The rheumatoid arthritis patients fulfilled the American College of Rheumatology criteria.

There were also 30 healthy controls individuals attending the blood bank in Helsinki.

The remainder of the serum samples were collected from two centres in Japan: 30 rheumatoid arthritis patients and 18 patients with systemic lupus erythematosus were attending the Rheumatology Department of the Juntendo University in Tokyo, as well as 23 serum samples taken from healthy individuals.

Another group of sera came from 30 rheumatoid arthritis patients in Otsu, from southern Japan and were provided by Dr. Yoshitaka Tani.

All Japanese rheumatoid arthritis patients were diagnosed according to the American Rheumatism Association criteria.

Synthetic Peptides and ELISA

The test and control peptides were prepared and synthesized by the solid phase method of Merrifield. Peptides were analysed for at least 90% purity by high-performance liquid chromatography as previously described.

For immunological studies, it is necessary to use 15–16 amino acid long sequences, because the terminal 3–4 amino acids will be in a random coil formation and only the central part of the peptide will be in an α-helix configuration.

Three 16-mer amino acid peptides prepared for this study included the following sequences:

1. SQKDLL**EQRRAA**VDTY which represents amino acid residues 63–78 contained within HLA-DR4/Dw 14 (DRB1*0404).

2. LGSIS**ESRRAL**QDSQR which represents amino acid residues 27–42 of *Proteus mirabilis* haemolysin (Hpmb).
3. LGSISRSELARQDSQR a control peptide which represents the same residues as the *Proteus mirabilis* haemolysin (Hpmb) containing the ESRRAL sequence but in a scrambled order.

ELISA studies were carried out as previously described.

Bacteria and Indirect Immunofluorescence Studies

Three microbes were included in the study: *Proteus mirabilis*, *Escherichia coli* and *Serratia marcescens*.

Measurement of bacterial antibodies by indirect immunofluorescence was carried out as previously described.

The end point was the last dilution showing definite fluorescence: no fluorescence at first dilution scored zero, fluorescence at first dilution = 1, fluorescence at second dilution = 2, and so on up to a maximum of 8 dilutions.

All sera were examined under code and in duplicate.

Bacterial Antibodies in Finnish Patients

Significantly elevated levels of *Proteus* IgG antibodies were found in both the 'Early rheumatoid arthritis' ($t = 4.10$, $p < 0.001$) and 'Advanced rheumatoid arthritis' ($t = 10.76$, $p < 0.001$) compared to healthy Finnish controls (Fig. 15.1).

Similar elevations were found in the *Proteus* IgM antibodies in both the 'Early rheumatoid arthritis' ($t = 2.28$, $p < 0.02$) and 'Advanced Rheumatoid arthritis' ($t = 9.85, p < 0.001$) compared to the corresponding healthy controls, but no such elevations were found in the IgA class.

By contrast, no significant immunoglobulin elevations were found against *Serratia marcescens* or *Escherichia coli* when compared to controls (Fig. 15.1).

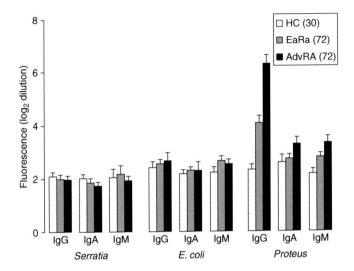

FIGURE 15.1 Bacterial isotypic antibodies (mean ± standard error) in Finnish patients with 'Early' (EaRA) and 'Advanced' (AdvRA) and Finnish healthy controls (HC) measured using indirect immunofluorescence (Reprinted with kind permission from Springer Science+Business Media, Rashid et al. (2004))

Bacterial Antibodies in Japanese Patients

Significant elevations in anti-*Proteus* IgG immunoglobulins were also observed among rheumatoid arthritis patients from Otsu ($t = 9.63$, $p < 0.001$) when compared to Japanese healthy controls or to Japanese patients with systemic lupus erythematosus ($t = 9.93$, $p < 0.001$) (Fig. 15.2).

Japanese rheumatoid arthritis patients from Tokyo also had elevated levels of anti-*Proteus* antibodies when compared to Japanese healthy controls ($t = 2.05$, $p < 0.05$) or to Japanese patients with systemic lupus erythematosus ($t = 2.89$, $p < 0.01$).

Furthermore there were also significant elevations in both anti-*Proteus* IgA ($t = 3.46$, $p < 0.005$) and IgM ($t = 2.78$, $p < 0.01$) antibodies in Otsu rheumatoid arthritis patients when compared to Japanese healthy controls.

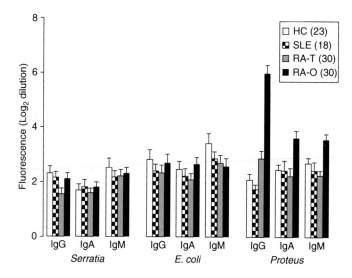

FIGURE 15.2 Bacterial isotypic antibodies (mean ± standard error) in Japanese patients with rheumatoid arthritis from Otsu (RA-O) or from Tokyo (RA-T), patients with systemic lupus erythematosus (SLE) and Japanese healthy controls (HC) measured by indirect immunofluorescence (Reprinted with kind permission from Springer Science+Business Media, Rashid et al. (2004))

By contrast, there were no significant antibody elevations against *Escherichia coli* or *Serratia marcescens*.

Antibodies to Peptides in Finnish Patients

Significant IgG antibody elevations were found against EQRRAA of HLA-DR1/4 in 'Early rheumatoid arthritis' ($t = 3.15$, $p < 0.005$) and 'Advanced rheumatoid arthritis' patients ($t = 8.17, p < 0.001$) when compared to healthy Finnish control subjects (Fig. 15.3).

There were also significant IgG antibody elevations against ESRRAL of *Proteus* haemolysin in 'Early

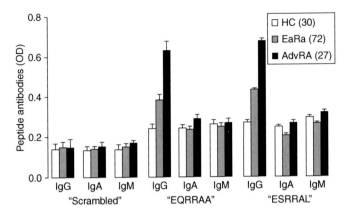

FIGURE 15.3 Peptide isotypic antibodies (mean ± standard error) in Finnish patients with 'Early' (EaRA) and 'Advanced' (AdvRA) and Finnish Healthy controls (HC) using ELISA (Reprinted with kind permission from Springer Science+Business Media, Rashid et al. (2004))

rheumatoid arthritis' ($t = 3.71$, $p < 0.001$) and 'Advanced rheumatoid arthritis' patients ($t = 8.05$, $p < 0.001$) when compared to healthy Finnish subjects.

By contrast, no significant difference was observed among any classes of immunoglobulins when 'Early rheumatoid arthritis' and 'Advanced rheumatoid arthritis' groups were compared to healthy Finnish subjects when tested with the control peptides (Fig. 15.3).

Antibodies to Peptides in Japanese Patients

Significant elevations in IgG immunoglobulins against EQRRAA of HLA-DR1/4 were also observed among rheumatoid arthritis patients from Otsu ($t = 7.68$, $p < 0.001$) when compared to Japanese healthy controls or to Japanese patients with systemic lupus erythematosus ($t = 6.86$, $p < 0.001$) (Fig. 15.4).

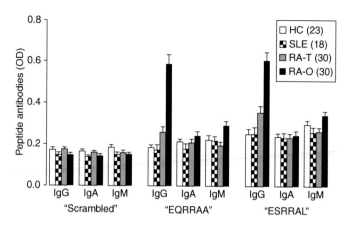

FIGURE 15.4 Peptide isotypic antibodies (mean ± standard error) in Japanese patients with rheumatoid arthritis from Otsu (RA-O) or from Tokyo (RA-T), patients with systemic lupus erythematosus (SLE) and Japanese healthy controls (HC) measured by ELISA (Reprinted with kind permission from Springer Science+Business Media, Rashid et al. (2004))

Moreover a significant elevation in immunoglobulins against EQRRAA of HLA-DR1/4 was also observed when rheumatoid arthritis patients from Tokyo were compared to healthy Japanese control subjects ($t = 2.30$, $p < 0.05$) or to Japanese patients with systemic lupus erythematosus ($t = 2.21$, $p < 0.05$).

Furthermore, significant elevations in immunoglobulins against ESRRAL of *Proteus mirabilis* were also observed among rheumatoid arthritis patients from Otsu when compared to Japanese healthy controls ($t = 7.68$, $p < 0.001$) or to Japanese patients with systemic lupus erythematosus ($t = 6.86$, $p < 0.001$) (Fig. 15.4). Moreover a significant elevation in IgG immunoglobulins against ESRRAL of *Proteus* haemolysin was also observed when rheumatoid arthritis patients from Tokyo were compared to healthy Japanese control subjects ($t = 2.49$, $p < 0.02$) or to Japanese patients with systemic lupus erythematosus ($t = 2.19$, $p < 0.05$).

However when determinations of other isotypes were carried out, increased antibody titres against EQRRAA ($t=2.55$, $p<0.02$) or ESRRAL ($t=2.60$, $p<0.02$) peptides were observed only among the IgM class of immunoglobulins and only in the Otsu group with rheumatoid arthritis compared to patients with systemic lupus erythematosus.

A significant difference was also observed in the IgM antibody level against the EQRRAA peptide of HLA-DR1/4 in the Otsu group of rheumatoid arthritis patients when compared to healthy Japanese controls ($t=2.92, p<0.01$).

By contrast, no significant differences were observed when the sera were screened against control peptides (Fig. 15.4).

Correlation Between Anti-*Proteus* Antibodies and Anti-Peptide Antibodies

There was a significant correlation when the total (IgG, IgM and IgA) antibody levels of both Finnish and Japanese patients were compared to the antibody levels of EQRRAA of HLA-DR1/4 ($r=0.79$, $p<0.001$) (Fig. 15.5a) and to the ESRRAL sequence of *Proteus* haemolysin ($r=0.86, p<0.001$) (Fig. 15.5b) but there was no correlation with antibodies to the other bacteria *Escherichia coli* or *Serratia marcescens* or to the control peptides.

Clinical Implications and Discussion

The results show increased antibodies are found only against *Proteus mirabilis* but not against two other microbes, *Escherichia coli* and *Serratia marcescens*, a remarkable observation since all three microbes carry in their primary structure the homologous rheumatoid arthritis susceptibility sequence or 'shared epitope'.

The study has shown that antibodies to *Proteus mirabilis* are present in Finnish patients or in Japanese patients coming from two different centres. The reason for the observation of

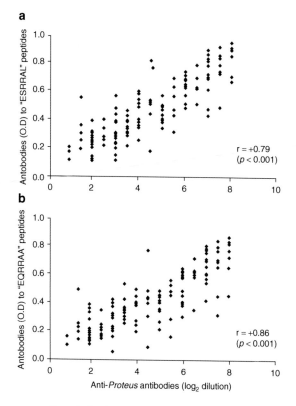

FIGURE 15.5 Correlation between total (IgG,IgA and IgM) antibodies and anti-peptide antibody levels in sera of Finnish and Japanese patients with rheumatoid arthritis ($n = 159$) (**a**) ESRRAL, (**b**) EQRRAA (Reprinted with kind permission from Springer Science+Business Media, Rashid et al. (2004))

higher antibody titres in the Otsu group compared to the Tokyo group could be due to a greater number of active patients being present in the Otsu group (Rashid et al. 2004).

These results are in agreement with those published from many other centres and raise issues as to the origin of this disease (Carty et al. 2003).

An HLA-DR4 association with rheumatoid arthritis has previously been reported in Japanese populations (Nakai et al. 1981).

It has been found that over 90% of rheumatoid arthritis patients belong to one of the HLA groups, DR1, DR4-Dw4 and DR4-Dw14, all of which contain the shared sequence EQ(K)RRAA or its homologue (Wallin et al. 1991).

The question arises whether the similarity or crossreactivity between the bacterial antigens and the self-antigens of the HLA group is sufficient or adequate to produce, in presence of complement, a cytotoxic activity by high titre of anti-*Proteus* antibodies whereby they could act as autoantibodies and cause tissue and joint damage.

References

Carty SM, Snowden M, Silman AJ. Should infection still be considered as the most likely triggering factor for rheumatoid arthritis ? J Rheumatol. 2003;30:425–9.

Nakai Y, Wakisaka A, Aizawa M, Itakura K, Nakai H, Ohashi A. HLA and rheumatoid arthritis in Japanese. Arthritis Rheum. 1981;24:722–5.

Rashid T, Leirisalo-Repo M, Tani Y, Hukuda S, Kobayashi S, Wilson C, et al. Antibacterial and antipeptide antibodies in Japanese and Finnish patients with rheumatoid arthritis. Clin Rheumatol. 2004;23:134–41.

Wallin J, Hillert J, Olerup O, Carlsson B, Strom H. Association of rheumatoid arthritis with a dominant DR1/Dw4, Dw14 sequence motif, but not with a T cell receptor β chain gene alleles or haplotypes. Arthritis Rheum. 1991;34:1416–24.

Chapter 16
Molecular Similarity Between the Rheumatoid Arthritis Associated Motif EQKRAA and Structurally Related Sequences of *Proteus*

Contents

A. Ebringer, *Rheumatoid Arthritis and Proteus*,
DOI 10.1007/978-0-85729-950-5_16,
© Springer-Verlag London Limited 2012

Introduction: The Association of the 'Shared Epitope' with Sequences of *Proteus* and Transfectant Cell Lines

The HLA-DR alleles, DRB1*0401, *0402, *0405, *0101 and *1402, which share an amino acid sequence EQR(K)RAA in the DRB1 chain, have been linked with a susceptibility to develop rheumatoid arthritis.

It has been suggested that an environmental factor interacting with a genetic predisposition contributes to the pathogenesis of rheumatoid arthritis and studies from our group have suggested that antigens present in the urinary microbe *Proteus mirabilis* are somehow involved in the pathology of this disease.

The mechanism by which the susceptibility motif predisposes to the disease is to some extent unknown, although the two main theories have been that the cavity of the 'shared epitope' presents as yet some unknown antigen to lymphocytes (Hammer et al. 1995) or the sequences making up the cavity share some 'molecular mimicry' with environmental agents such as the urinary microbe *Proteus mirabilis* (Wilson et al. 2000).

Our studies were undertaken to determine the extent of cross-reactivity between the rheumatoid arthritis associated motifs **EQKRAA** and **EQRRAA** with the non-rheumatoid arthritis associated motif **EDERAA** and compare them to the *Proteus mirabilis* bacterial haemolysin sequence **ESRRAL**.

Peptide Synthesis

The peptides were assembled by using an automated Milligen Biosearch model 9050 Pepsynthesizer on NovaSyn TG flow resin with a loading value of 0.41 mmol·g/l, functionalized with a Rink amide linker. Acylation cycles with (four equivalents) Fmoc (9-fluorenylmethoxycarbonyl) amino acid, preactivated with 2(1-H-benzo-triazo-1-yl)-1,1,9-tetramethyl uranium tetrafluoroborate (TBTU) and di-iso-propyl-ethylamine (DIPEA) in a molar ratio (1:1:1.5 by volume) were carried out in DMF for 30–40 min. Fmoc deprotection was achieved with 20% piperidine in DMF. N-terminal acetylation was carried out by using pentafluorophenyl acetate (4 equivalents)for 30 min. Reactions were monitored by UV detection of the column effluent at 365 nm and colour tests for free amino groups (Kaiser et al. 1980). Complete peptidyl resins were washed successively with DMF, methanol and diethyl ether before being dried in vacuo. The peptidyl resin was treated with a solution (10 ml) of trifluoroacetic acid (TFA)-H_2O-tri-iso-propyl-silane (94:5:1 by volume) for 90 min at room temperature. The resin was then filtered through a sintered funnel and washed with TFA, and the combined filtrate was dried by rotary evaporation. Residual TFA was azeotroped with diethyl ether. The products were lyophilized from water and purified by preparative high-performance liquid chromatography with a Vidac 218TP54 column on a Waters 900 photodiode array system. Solvent A was 0.1% TFA and solvent B was 10% solvent A plus 90% acetonitrile. All peptides used had a purity in excess of 90% and their masses were determined by using a Bioanalysis MALDI-TOF instrument with a-cyano-4-hydroxycinnamic acid as the matrix.

The molecular mimicry sequences are shown in bold. The sequences of the peptides were as follows:

1. The HLA-DRB1*0401 peptide, CKDLL**EQRRAA**VDTYC (residues 65–79) which is associated with rheumatoid arthritis.
2. The HLA-DRB1*0402 peptide, CKDIL**EDERAA**VDTYC (residues 65–79) which is NOT associated with rheumatoid arthritis.
3. The *Proteus mirabilis* haemolysin peptide, CLGSIS-**ESRRAL**QDSQR (residues 27–42).

A cysteine residue was attached to all three peptides at the N terminus for coupling of the synthetic peptide to the carrier protein.

Peptide Antisera

Synthetic peptides of HLA-DRB1*0401, HLA-DRB1*0402 and *Proteus mirabilis* haemolysin sequence were conjugated to the carrier protein keyhole limpet haemocyanin (KLH) (ICN Biomedical Ltd) by using m-maleiimido-benzoyl-N-hydroxysuccinimide ester (Green et al. 1982).

The conjugate was purified by gel filtration with PD10 columns (Sigma Chemical Ltd.). New Zealand White rabbits received three subcutaneous injections at 2-week intervals. A 250 µl of a 1 mg/ml solution (synthetic peptide conjugated to KLH) was added to 250 µl of Specol adjuvant (Central Veterinary Institute). Peptide antiserum reactivity was continuously monitored by measuring the immune response to various concentrations of both the target peptide and KLH alone. The rabbits were bled 14 days after the last immunisation, and the resultant sera were stored at –20°C.

ELISA

Antibody responses were measured by peptide enzyme-linked-immunosorbent assay (ELISA) as previously described.

For inhibition studies, the inhibitors, KDLL**EQKRAA**-VDTYC, LGSIS**ESRRAL**QDSQR and KDIL**EDERAA** (100 µg/ml), were incubated overnight at 37°C with the three peptide antisera, before ELISAs were carried out. All ELISAs were carried out in triplicate, and the mean OD value (± standard error) was calculated for each sample.

Mouse Fibroblast (Dap 3) Cells

Mouse fibroblast Dap.3 cells transfected with HLA-DRB1*0401, HLA-DRB1*0402 and untransfected cells, together with L243 (anti-DRα) in supernatant form, were kindly provided by Prof. R. Lechler of the Department of Immunology, Hammersmith Hospital, London, England.

Both sets of transfected and untransfected cells were maintained as previously described (Barber et al. 1991). However, transfected cells were also grown in the presence of G418 (200 μl/ml) (Gibco). The formation of an adherent monolayer indicates healthy growth.

Dilution Studies with Peptide Antisera

The results obtained in this study demonstrate cross-reactivity between KDLL**EQKRAA**VDTYC and LGSIS**ESRRAL** but not with the Dw 10 motif KDIL**EDERAA**VDTYC when tested by ELISA.

Increased binding activity by the HLA-DRB1*0401 peptide antiserum and the *Proteus mirabilis* haemolysin peptide antiserum was present compared to the HLA-DRB1*0402 peptide antiserum.

The mean optical density (OD) (± standard error) at a dilution of 1/1,600 of the DRB1*0401 peptide antiserum tested against the *Proteus mirabilis* haemolysin peptide was 0.87 ± 0.02 OD units which was significantly higher than the value of 0.11 ± 0.03 OD units obtained for binding with the DRB1*0402 peptide antiserum or the value of 0.02 ± 0.02 OD units obtained with the pre-immune serum (Fig. 16.1).

Furthermore the DRB1*0401 antiserum bound to the *Proteus mirabilis* haemolysin peptide up to a dilution of 1/51,200, while DRB1*0402 antiserum stopped reacting at 1/6,400 (Fig. 16.1).

Binding activity of the *Proteus mirabilis* haemolysin peptide antiserum and the DRB1*0401 peptide antiserum was increased compared to the DRB1*0402 peptide antiserum.

The mean (± standard error) OD units binding at 1/1,600 dilution of the *Proteus mirabilis* peptide antiserum was 0.77 ± 0.04 OD units which was significantly higher than the value of 0.05 ± 0.02 OD units obtained for the DRB1*0402 peptide antiserum or the value of 0.04 ± 0.01 OD units obtained with the pre-immune serum (Fig. 16.2).

The *Proteus mirabilis* haemolysin peptide antiserum bound to DRB1*0401 peptide at 1/25,600, whereas the DRB1*0402 peptide antiserum reacted at dilutions of up to 1/6,400 (Fig. 16.2).

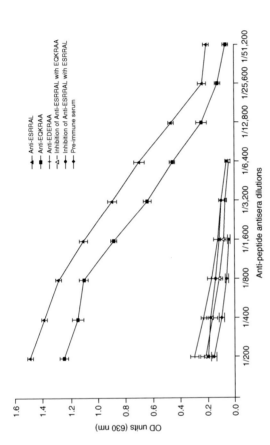

FIGURE 16.1 Anti-peptide antiserum dilutions response curves with ELISA. The antisera were raised against the following KLH conjugates of peptide CKDLLEQKRAAVDTYC, CLGSISESRRALQDSQR and CKDILEDERAAVDTYC. The binding of the antisera and pre-immune serum was determined by using the uncoupled peptide LGSISESRRALQDSQR adsorbed onto the ELISA plate. Also shown is the inhibition by the indicated peptide (With permission from Tiwana et al. (1999))

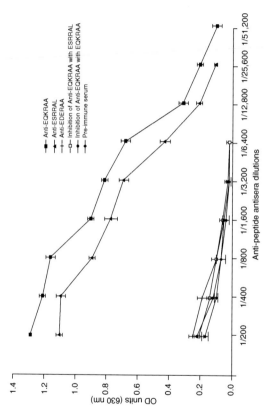

FIGURE 16.2 Anti-peptide antiserum dilutions response curves with ELISA. The antisera were raised against the following KLH conjugates of peptide CKDLLEE**QKRAA**VDTYC, CLGSISES**RRAL**QDSQR and CKDILE**DERAA**VDTYC. The binding of the antisera and pre-immune serum was determined by using the uncoupled peptide KDLLEE**QKRAA** VDTYC adsorbed onto the ELISA plate. Also shown is the inhibition by the indicated peptide (With permission from Tiwana et al. (1999))

However, there was no increased binding activity between DRB1*0401 and *Proteus mirabilis* haemolysin peptide antisera, respectively to DRB1*0402 (Fig. 16.3).

Furthermore, there was no reactivity to keyhole limpet haemocyanin (KLH) when all three peptide antiserum samples were tested.

Inhibition Studies

Peptide antiserum raised against DRB1*0401 was inhibited by pre-incubation with 100 µg of LGSIS**ESRRAL**QDSQR peptide per ml, as well as with KDLL**EQKRRA**VDTYC peptide.

In a similar way, antisera raised against the *Proteus mirabilis* haemolysin sequence was also inhibited by preincubation with 100 µg/ml of KDLL**EQKRAA**VDTYC (Fig. 16.1) or preincubation with 100 µg/ml of LGSIS**ESRRAL**QDSQR (Fig. 16.2).

The anti-CLGSIS**ESRRAL**QDSQR antiserum prior to incubation with DRB1*0401 peptide had a mean (± standard error) antibody-binding activity of 1.49 ± 0.02 OD units at a dilution of 1/200 and reacted at dilutions of up to 1/51,200. After incubation, the binding activity was reduced to 0.20 ± 0.04 at a dilution of 1/200 and reacted at dilutions up to 1/6,400.

Similar results were obtained with LGSIS**ESRRAL**QDSQR peptide. The DRB1*0401 antiserum had a mean (± standard error) to the DRB1*0401 peptide of 1.29 ± 0.01 OD units at 1/200 dilution and bound up to a dilution of 1/51,200.

However, after incubation with the LGSIS**ESRRAL**QDSQR peptide, the peptide activity was reduced to 0.21 ± 0.02 at 1/200 dilution and the serum reacted at a dilution of 1/6,400 (Fig. 16.2).

Furthermore, similar results were obtained with the KDLL**EQRRAA**VDTYC peptide (Fig. 16.2).

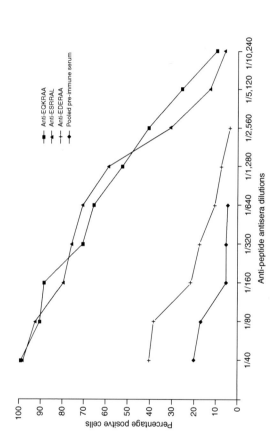

FIGURE 16.4 Dilution studies of antisera raised against CKDLLEQKRAAVDTYC, CLGSISESRRALQDSQR and CKDILEDERAAVDTYC peptides and pooled pre-immune rabbit serum binding to mouse fibroblast transfected cell line Dap.3 expressing HLA-DRB1*0401 (DR4/Dw4). The percentage of cells which fluoresce at levels greater than the arbitrarily set level of 10^1 are shown (With permission from Tiwana et al. (1999))

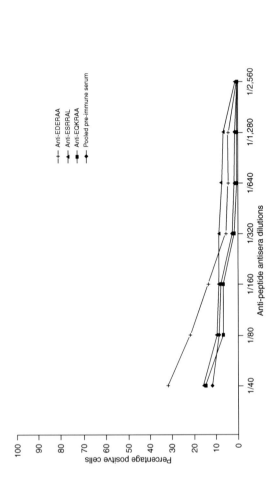

FIGURE 16.5 Dilution studies of antisera raised to **CKDLLEQKRAA**VDTYC, CLGSISES**RRA**LQDSQR and CKDIL**EDERAA**VDTYC peptides and pooled pre-immune serum binding to the mouse fibroblast transfected cell line Dap.3 expressing HLA-DRB1*0402 (DR4/Dw10). The percentage of cells which fluoresce at levels greater than the arbitrarily set level of 10^1 are shown (With permission from Tiwana et al. (1999))

In a reciprocal manner, antisera raised against the *Proteus mirabilis* haemolysin sequence demonstrated greater binding affinity towards the rheumatoid arthritis susceptibility motif than the EDERAA peptide sequence of HLA-DRB1*0402 found in the HLA-Dw10 complex, an allele not associated with rheumatoid arthritis.

The results presented in this study suggest that antibodies raised against *Proteus mirabilis* ESRRAL antigens during urinary tract infections could possible bind, albeit with lower affinity, to HLA-DR4-positive cells in tissues expressing the class II HLA antigens EQKRAA and EQRRAA, fix complement and so initiate local inflammation that could lead to destruction of self-tissues in the joints by antibody-dependent cell cytotoxicity (Tiwana et al. 1999).

References

Barber LD, Bal V, Lamb JR, O'Hehir J, Yendle J, Hancock RJT, et al. Contribution of T-cell receptor contacting and peptide binding residues of the class II molecules of HLA-DR4.Dw10 to serologic and antigen specific T-cell recognition. Hum Immunol. 1991;32:110–8.

Green N, Alexander H, Olson A, Alexander S, Shinnick TM, Sutcliffe JG, et al. Immunogenic structure of the influenza virus haemagglutinin. Cell. 1982;28:477–87.

Hammer J, Gallazzi F, Bono E, Karr RW, Guenot J, Valsasnini P, et al. Peptide binding specificity of HLA-DR4 molecules: correlation with rheumatoid arthritis association. J Exp Med. 1995;181:1847–55.

Kaiser E, Bossinger CD, Colescott RL, Olsen DB. Colour test for terminal proline residues in solid phase synthesis of peptides. Ann Chem Acta. 1980;118:149–51.

Tiwana H, Wilson C, Alvarez A, Abuknesha R, Bansal S, Ebringer A. Cross-reactivity between the rheumatoid arthritis associated motif EQKRAA and structurally related sequences found in *Proteus mirabilis*. Infect Immun. 1999;67:2769–75.

Wilson C, Tiwana H, Ebringer A. Molecular mimicry between HLA-DR alleles associated with rheumatoid arthritis and *Proteus mirabilis* as the aetiological basis for autoimmunity. Microbes Infect. 2000;2:1489–96.

Chapter 17
Rheumatoid Arthritis Sera Are Cytotoxic to Cells Bearing HLA and Collagen Susceptibility Sequences

Contents

A. Ebringer, *Rheumatoid Arthritis and Proteus*,
DOI 10.1007/978-0-85729-950-5_17,
© Springer-Verlag London Limited 2012

Introduction: The Association of the 'Shared Epitope' EQ(R)RAA with the ESRRAL Sequence of *Proteus* Haemolysin and the Link of *Proteus* Urease with Collagen

The HLA-DR alleles, DRB1*0401, *0402, *0405, *0101 and *1402, which share an amino acid sequence EQR(K)RAA in the DRB1 chain, have been linked with a susceptibility to develop rheumatoid arthritis.

It has been suggested that an environmental factor interacting with a genetic predisposition contributes to the pathogenesis of rheumatoid arthritis.

We have reported that rheumatoid arthritis patients with active disease have elevated levels of antibodies to the urinary microbe *Proteus mirabilis* and this has been confirmed by several independent groups, such as one in the UK (Senior et al. 1995) and another one in the USA (Newkirk et al. 2005).

The level of anti-*Proteus* antibodies correlates with urinary isolation rates of *Proteus mirabilis* from patients with active rheumatoid arthritis.

Amino acid homologies and immunological crossreactivity between the susceptibility motif EQR(K)RAA and *Proteus mirabilis* haemolysin ESRRAL as well as type XI collagen LRREI and *Proteus mirabilis* urease IRRET have been demonstrated in studies from the Immunology Unit at King's College in London.

   Ankylosing spondylitis is a chronic inflammatory disorder affecting predominantly the lumbar spine and where 95% of patients are HLA-B27-positive. Increased levels of antibodies to the gut microbe *Klebsiella pneumoniae* have been reported, suggesting an aetiological role for this microbe in the pathogenesis of this disease. Sera from patients with this condition have been used as 'disease controls' for these cytotoxicity studies in patients with rheumatoid arthritis.

   Amino acid sequence homologies have been identified between HLA-B*2705 (QTDRED) and two enzymes present in *Klebsiella pneumoniae*, nitrogenase reductase (QTDRED) and pullulanase secretion protein pul D (DRDE) (Fielder et al. 1995).

   Patients with active ankylosing spondylitis have been shown to have elevated levels of antibodies to all three peptide sequences compared to control groups.

   The cytotoxic activity of sera from rheumatoid arthritis patients and ankylosing spondylitis has been investigated to determine whether tissue-damaging properties were present in patients when compared to sera obtained from healthy individuals.

Sera from Rheumatoid Arthritis and Ankylosing Spondylitis Patients

Sera were collected from patients with active rheumatoid arthritis, (erythrocyte sedimentation rate > 15 mm/h) attending the Department of Rheumatology at the Lister Hospital in Stevenage and ankylosing spondylitis patients attending the 'Ankylosing Spondylitis Research Clinic' of the Middlesex Hospital in London.

   The diagnosis of rheumatoid arthritis was made according to the American Rheumatism Criteria and the diagnosis of ankylosing spondylitis was made according to the New York criteria.

   Antibodies against synthetic peptides 15-/16-mer peptides containing ESRRAL, EQRRAA, LRREI, IRRET, EDERAA,

QTDRED and DRED as well as control sequences were measured in the sera obtained from rheumatoid arthritis and ankylosing spondylitis patients.

There were 51 patients with rheumatoid arthritis, 18 men and 33 women with a mean age of 49 years (range: 28–70 years). Their mean (± standard error) erythrocyte sedimentation rate was 45.4 ± 9.6 mm/h.

There were 34 patients with ankylosing spondylitis, 26 men and 8 women with a mean age of 46 years (range: 23–69 years). Their mean (± standard error) erythrocyte sedimentation rate was 48.2 ± 3.7 mm/h.

Sera were also obtained from 38 healthy blood donors, 18 men and 28 women with a mean age of 40 years (range: 24–57 years).

Synthetic Peptides and ELISA

Peptides were prepared by solid phase synthesis and analysed for purity by high-performance liquid chromatography as previously described. All peptides had at least 90% purity. The molecular mimicry sequences are shown in bold.

The test peptides were:

1. SQKDLL**EQRRAA**VDTY of HLA-DRB1*0404
2. LGSS**ESRRAL**QDSQR of *Proteus mirabilis* haemolysin
3. QSLDS**LRREI**EQMRR of type XI collagen
4. FAESR**IRRET**IAAED of *Proteus mirabilis* urease
5. Control peptide SQKDIL**EDERAA**VDTY of HLA-DRB1*0402
6. CKAKA**QTDRED**LRTLL of HLA-B*2705
7. RPTVIR**DRDE**YRQASS of *Klebsiella pneumoniae* pullulanase
8. ASLEHEEGKILRAQLE of human myosin
9. KKLTEKEAELQAKLE of *Streptococcus pyogenes*
10. LGSISRSELARQDSQR of scrambled haemolysin
11. RPTVRSDIDYRQAESR of scrambled pullulanase

The ELISA was carried out as previously described.

All assays were carried out in duplicate and under code, so that the status of each serum sample under investigation was not known to the tester.

Preparation of Sheep Red Blood Cells for Cytotoxicity Assay

A 20-ml aliquot of sheep blood (Unipath Ltd, Hampshire, UK) was washed twice with 0.85% sodium chloride (saline) solution in a centrifuge (Heraeus, minifuge) at 750 × g (3,000 rpm) for 15 min. Supernatant was discarded, and 600 µl of the packed cells were removed and placed into each of two universal containers. The cells in each container were resuspended in 10 ml saline and 10 ml of a 1/20,000 tannic acid (Aldrich Chemical Co, Dover, UK) in saline added to each container, followed by mixing and incubation for 15 min at 37°C in a water bath. After centrifugation for 5 min, the supernatant was discarded and cells resuspended in 20-ml saline and washed. One container was later used as a negative control.

The cells in the other container were resuspended in 10-ml saline and 10-ml antigen (2 mg/ml) added, followed by mixing and incubation for 30 min at 37°C in a water bath. After washing by centrifugation for 5 min, the supernatant was discarded, the cells were washed 3 times with saline and both coated and uncoated (Control) cells resuspended in 50 ml of saline.

Serum samples were inactivated in a water bath at 56°C for 30 min.

The cytotoxicity assay was carried out as follows: 100 ml of serum diluted 1/8 in saline was added to 96 well microtitre plates (Dynatech) together with 100 µl of peptide-coated sheep red blood cells and the plates incubated at 37°C for 30 min. A 100-µl aliquot of guinea pig complement (Calbiochem Ltd., Nottingham, UK) diluted 1/10 in saline was added followed by mixing, then incubated at 37°C for 30 min and later at 4°C overnight to allow the unlysed cells to settle.

A 100-µl aliquot of test supernatant was removed and placed into wells of a microtitre plate and absorbance measured 570 nm.

Minimum lysis was calculated from peptide-coated cells treated with saline plus complement, and absorbance value obtained from the minimum lysis was subtracted from each test value. One hundred percent lysis was calculated from

100 μl of uncoated cells treated with 200 μl of distilled water and this was labelled as 'maximum lysis'.

Percentage lysis was determined using the following formula:

$$\%\text{Lysis} = \frac{\left(\text{Test lysis} - \text{minimum lysis}\right)}{\left(\text{Maximum lysis} - \text{minimum lysis}\right)} \times 100$$

All assays were carried in duplicate and under code, in that the tester did not know which sera came from patients or control subjects.

Antibody Absorption Assay

Serum samples from five rheumatoid arthritis patients with high antibody levels to the individual peptides were absorbed with 250 μl of packed sheep red blood cells coated with ESRRAL, EQRRAA, IRRET and LRREI peptide sequences in a plastic tube overnight at 4°C, with gentle rotation. The absorption process was repeated until the antibody level for each sample was below the mean value of the control subjects, measured by ELISA.

The absorbed sera were then tested for cytotoxic activity against sheep red blood cells coated with EQRRAA and LRREI peptides, as described above.

Antibodies to Peptide Antigens in Rheumatoid Arthritis Patients

HLA-DRB1*0404 Peptide

The levels of IgG antibodies to the HLA-DRB1*0404 peptide SQKDLL**EQRRAA**VDTY of the IgG class were significantly elevated in rheumatoid arthritis patients when compared to ankylosing spondylitis patients or healthy controls. The mean

(± standard error) level in rheumatoid arthritis patients was 0.537 ± 0.013 OD units and this was significantly higher than the level of 0.134 ± 0.006 OD units found in ankylosing spondylitis patients ($t=23.65, p<0.0001$) or the level of 0.152 ± 0.010 OD units found in healthy controls ($t=21.62, p<0.0001$).

There was no significant difference between ankylosing spondylitis patients and healthy controls when tested against the DRB1*0404 peptide.

Proteus mirabilis Haemolysin Peptide

The levels of IgG antibodies to the *Proteus mirabilis* haemolysin peptide LGSIS**ESRRAL**QDSQR were significantly elevated in rheumatoid arthritis patients when compared to ankylosing spondylitis patients or healthy controls. The mean (± standard error) level in rheumatoid arthritis patients was 0.590 ± 0.015 OD units and this was significantly higher than the level of 0.155 ± 0.008 OD units found in ankylosing spondylitis patients ($t=22.17, p<0.0001$) or the level of 0.170 ± 0.010 found in healthy controls ($t=21.38, p<0.0001$). There was no significant difference between ankylosing spondylitis patients and healthy controls when tested against the *Proteus mirabilis* haemolysin peptide.

Type XI Collagen Peptide

The levels of IgG antibodies to the type XI collagen peptide GSLD**LRREI**EQMRR were significantly elevated in rheumatoid arthritis patients when compared to the ankylosing spondylitis or healthy controls. The mean (± standard error) level in rheumatoid arthritis patients was 0.490 ± 0.009 OD units, and this was significantly higher than the level of 0.133 ± 0.007 OD units found in ankylosing spondylitis patients ($t=30.08, p<0.0001$) or the level of 0.136 ± 0.007 OD units found in healthy controls ($t=26.17, p<0.0001$).

There was no significant difference between the ankylosing spondylitis patients and healthy controls when tested against the type XI collagen peptide.

Proteus mirabilis Urease Peptide

The levels of IgG antibodies to the *Proteus mirabilis* urease peptide FAESR**IRRET**IAAED were significantly elevated in rheumatoid arthritis patients when compared to ankylosing spondylitis patients or healthy controls. The mean (± standard error) in rheumatoid arthritis patients was 0.514 ± 0.010 OD units and this was significantly higher than the level of 0.146 ± 0.007 OD units found in ankylosing spondylitis patients ($t = 26.13$, $p < 0.0001$) or the level of 0.171 ± 0.012 OD units found in healthy controls ($t = 22.0, p < 0.0001$).

There was no significant difference between the ankylosing spondylitis patients and healthy controls when tested against the *Proteus mirabilis* urease peptide.

DRB1*0402 Peptide

There was no significant reactivity (mean ± standard error) to the DRB1*0402 peptide SQDIL**EDERAA**VDTY in the two groups of patients, rheumatoid arthritis (0.132 ± 0.007) or ankylosing spondylitis (0.113 ± 0.008), when compared to healthy blood donor subjects (0.131 ± 0.009).

Cytotoxicity Studies in Rheumatoid Arthritis Patients

Sera from rheumatoid arthritis and ankylosing spondylitis patients as well as sera from healthy blood donors were tested for reactivity in a complement-mediated cytotoxicity assay with sheep red blood cells coated with HLA.DRB1*0402

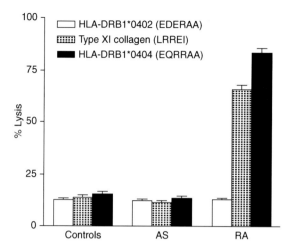

FIGURE 17.1 Percentage lysis of sheep *red* blood cells coated with HLA-DRB1*0404 (*EQRRAA*), DRB1*0402 (*EDERAA*) and type XI collagen (*LRREI*) peptides, via complement-mediated cytotoxicity by control sera and sera from ankylosing spondylitis (*AS*) rheumatoid arthritis (*RA*) patients (With kind permission from Wilson et al. (2003))

(EDERAA) peptide, type XI collagen (LRREI) peptide and HLA-DRB1*0404 (EQRRAA) peptide (Fig. 17.1).

EQRRAA Peptide

The sera from rheumatoid arthritis patients showed significantly higher levels of cytotoxic activity against sheep red blood cells coated with SQKDLL**EQRRAA**VDTY from HLA-DRB1*0404 when compared to ankylosing spondylitis patients or healthy controls. The mean (± standard error) percentage lysis in rheumatoid arthritis patients was $83.3 \pm 2.2\%$ and this was significantly higher than the level $13.7 \pm 0.8\%$ found in ankylosing spondylitis patients ($t = 25.63, p < 0.0001$) or the level of $15.5 \pm 1.2\%$ ($t = 25.06, p < 0.0001$) found in healthy controls.

There was no significant difference in the cytotoxic activity of the ankylosing spondylitis sera or the ones obtained from healthy controls, when tested against sheep red blood cells coated with the HLA-DRB1*0404 (EQRRAA) peptide.

LRREI Peptide

The sera from rheumatoid arthritis patients showed significantly higher levels of cytotoxic activity against sheep red blood cells coated with GSLDS**LRREI**EQMRR from type XI collagen when compared to ankylosing spondylitis patients or healthy controls.

The mean (± standard error) percentage lysis in rheumatoid arthritis patients was $65.7 \pm 2.2\%$, and this was significantly higher than the level of $11.5 \pm 0.9\%$ found in ankylosing spondylitis patients ($t = 19.16$, $p < 0.0001$) or the level of $13.7 \pm 1.3\%$ found in healthy controls ($t = 18.43$, $p < 0.0001$).

There was no significant difference in the cytotoxic activity of the ankylosing spondylitis sera or the ones obtained from healthy controls when tested against sheep red blood cells coated with the type XI collagen peptide.

EDERAA Peptide

There was no significant cytotoxic reactivity against sheep red blood cells coated with SQKDIL**EDERAA**VDTY of HLA-DRB1*0402 in the rheumatoid arthritis or ankylosing spondylitis sera when compared to sera from healthy blood donors.

Correlation Between ESRRAL and IRRET Antibodies

There was a significant correlation between anti-*Proteus mirabilis* haemolysin peptide (ESRRAL) antibodies and percentage lysis of sheep red blood cells coated with SQKDLL**EQRRAA**VDTY of HLA-DR1*0404 ($r = 0.970$, $p < 0.0001$) (Fig. 17.2a).

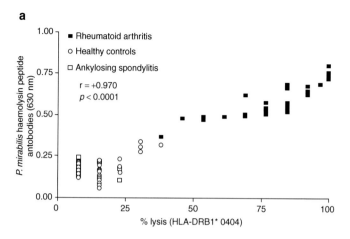

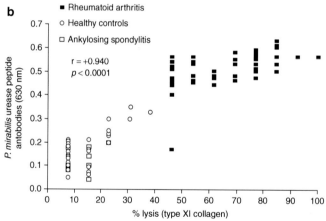

FIGURE 17.2 Correlation of anti-*Proteus mirabilis*haemolysin (**a**) and anti-*Proteus mirabilis*urease (**b**) IgG antibody levels for rheumatoid arthritis and ankylosing spondylitis patients and healthy controls and percentage lysis of sheep *red*blood cells coated with HLA-DRB1*0404 and type XI collagen peptides respectively (With kind permission from Wilson et al. (2003))

There was also a significant correlation between anti-*Proteus mirabilis* urease (IRRET) and percentage lysis of sheep red blood cells coated with GSLDS**LRREI**EQMRR of type XI collagen ($r = 0.940$, $p < 0.0001$) (Fig. 17.2b).

Furthermore, there was also a significant correlation between anti-EQRRAA antibodies and percentage lysis of sheep red blood cells coated with EQRRAA peptide ($r = 0.954$, $p < 0.0001$).

There also was a significant correlation between anti-IRRET antibodies and sheep red blood cells coated with IRRET peptide ($r = 0.948$, $p < 0.0001$).

Results of Absorption Studies

Absorbed sera from 5 rheumatoid arthritis patients were tested for reactivity in complement-mediated cytotoxicity with sheep red blood cells coated with EQRRAA and LRREI peptides.

The mean percentage lysis of sheep red blood cells coated with EQRRAA peptide was 100%.

The mean percentage lysis of sheep red blood coated with LRREI peptides was 82%.

However, after absorption with sheep red blood cells coated with EQRRAA or ESRRAL, the mean percentage lysis was 13.7%.

Furthermore, after absorption with sheep red blood cells coated with LRREI or IRRET peptides, it was 12.2% (Table 17.1).

Absorption analyses with EQRRAA, ESRRAL, LRREI and IRRET thus resulted in the reduction of percentage lysis.

Antibodies to Peptide Antigens in Ankylosing Spondylitis Patients

Levels of IgG antibodies to the HLA-B27 peptide CKAKAQ**QTDRED**LRTLL in ankylosing spondylitis patients were significantly elevated compared to rheumatoid arthritis patients and healthy blood donor controls.

Table 17.1 Antibody absorption assay on 5 rheumatoid arthritis sera

Absorbing test peptides	ELISA (OD units)		Percentage LYSIS (%)	
	Pre-absorption	Post-absorption	Pre-absorption	Post-absorption
HLA-DRB1 *0404	0.63 ± 0.005	0.13 ± 0.009	100 ± 0.0	13.7 ± 1.4
P. mirabilis haemolysin	0.72 ± 0.004	0.11 ± 0.010	ND	ND
Type XI collagen	0.56 ± 0.009	0.12 ± 0.007	82.4 ± 4.2	12.2 ± 1.7
P. mirabilis urease	0.59 ± 0.010	0.13 ± 0.010	ND	ND

The mean ± standard error of the absorbance values (630 nm) and the percentage lysis are given
ND not done

The mean (± standard error) in ankylosing spondylitis patients was 0.491 ± 0.011 OD units and this was significantly greater than the level of 0.181 ± 0.012 OD units found in rheumatoid arthritis patients ($t=18.52, p<0.0001$) or the level of 0.223 ± 0.015 OD units ($t=14.15, p<0.0001$) found in healthy controls.

There was no significant difference in the level of antibodies to the HLA-B27 peptide between rheumatoid arthritis patients and healthy blood donors.

Levels of IgG antibodies to the *Klebsiella pneumoniae* nitrogenase peptide CNSR**QTDRED**ELIIA were significantly elevated in ankylosing spondylitis patients compared to rheumatoid arthritis patients and healthy blood donors.

The mean (± standard error) in ankylosing spondylitis patients was 0.529 ± 0.011 OD units and this was significantly greater than the level of 0.197 ± 0.012 OD units found in rheumatoid arthritis patients ($t=18.89, p<0.0001$) or the level of 0.233 ± 0.014 OD units ($t=15.96, p<0.0001$) found in healthy controls.

There was no significant difference in the level of antibodies to the *Klebsiella pneumoniae* nitrogenase peptide between rheumatoid arthritis patients and healthy blood donors.

Levels of IgG antibodies to the *Klebsiella pneumoniae* pullulanase peptide RPTVIR**DRDE**YRQASS were significantly elevated in ankylosing spondylitis patients compared to rheumatoid arthritis and healthy blood donors.

The mean (± standard error) in ankylosing spondylitis patients was 0.530 ± 0.010 OD units and this was significantly greater than the level of 0.183 ± 0.012 OD units found in rheumatoid arthritis patients ($t = 20.15$, $p < 0.0001$) or the level of 0.218 ± 0.016 OD units ($t = 16.32$, $p < 0.0001$) found in healthy controls.

There was no significant difference in the level of antibodies to the *Klebsiella pneumoniae* pullulanase peptide between rheumatoid arthritis patients and healthy blood donors.

There was no significant reactivity of rheumatoid arthritis and ankylosing spondylitis sera when compared to the sera from healthy blood donors to the following peptides from: human myosin, *Streptococcus pyogenes* and the scrambled peptides from haemolysin or pullulanase.

Cytotoxicity Studies in Ankylosing Spondylitis Patients

Sera from ankylosing spondylitis and rheumatoid arthritis patients, as well as sera from healthy controls were tested for complement-mediated cytotoxicity against sheep red cells coated with HLA-B27*2705 synthetic peptide.

The sera from ankylosing spondylitis patients showed significantly higher percentage lysis for sheep red blood cells coated with CKAKA**QTDRED**LRTLL of HLA.B*2705 peptide when compared to rheumatoid arthritis patients or healthy controls (Fig. 17.3).

The mean (± standard error) percentage lysis in ankylosing spondylitis patients was $69.2 \pm 3.1\%$ and this was significantly higher than the level found in rheumatoid arthritis patients which was $14.8 \pm 1.1\%$ ($t = 19.28$, $p < 0.0001$) or the level of $16.3 \pm 1.4\%$ ($t = 16.13$, $p < 0.0001$) found in healthy blood donors.

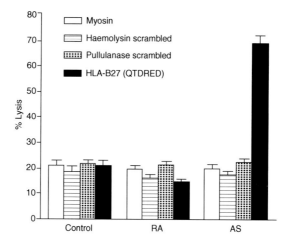

FIGURE 17.3 Percentage lysis of sheep *red* blood cells coated with HLA-B27 peptide (*QTDRED*) and other peptides via complement-mediated cytotoxicity by control sera and sera from patients with rheumatoid arthritis (*RA*) and ankylosing spondylitis (*AS*) (With kind permission from Wilson et al. (2003))

There was no significant difference in the cytotoxic activity of rheumatoid arthritis sera or the ones obtained from healthy donors when tested against sheep red blood cells coated with the HLA-B*2705 peptide.

No significant differences were found between ankylosing spondylitis and rheumatoid arthritis patients or healthy controls when testing sheep red blood cells coated with either human myosin, haemolysin scrambled or pullulanase scrambled peptides.

Correlation Between Cytotoxicity and Antibodies

There was a significant correlation between anti-nitrogenase antibodies and percentage lysis of sheep red blood cells coated with HLA-B*2705 (QTDRED) peptides for the ankylosing spondylitis and rheumatoid arthritis as well as the healthy control subjects ($r = +0.826, p < 0.0001$) (Fig. 17.4a).

There was also a significant correlation between anti-pullulanase (DRDE) antibodies and percentage lysis of sheep red blood cells coated with HLA-B*2705 (QTDRED) peptide for the ankylosing spondylitis and rheumatoid arthritis patients as well as the healthy control subjects ($r = +0.823, p < 0.0001$) (Fig. 17.4b).

There was also a significant correlation between anti-HLA-B*2705 antibodies and percentage lysis of sheep red blood cells coated with HLA-B*2705 (QTDRED) peptide for the ankylosing spondylitis and rheumatoid arthritis patients as well as the healthy control subjects ($r = +0.817, p < 0.0001$).

Discussion and Conclusions

Rheumatoid arthritis patients have been shown to have increased levels of antibodies against synthetic peptides derived from *Proteus mirabilis* haemolysin (ESRRAL), HLA-DRB*0404 (EQRRAA), type XI collagen (LRREI) and *Proteus mirabilis* urease (IRRET).

However, we were unable to find any significant increase in levels of antibodies to HLA-DRB1*0402 (EDERAA) peptide, a histocompatibility group not linked to rheumatoid arthritis.

These findings confirm our previous reports and those of others that rheumatoid arthritis patients have increased levels of antibodies against synthetic peptides containing ESRRAL (Dybwad et al. 1996) and EQRRAA (Takeuchi et al. 1990) sequences.

Further, rheumatoid arthritis sera are cytotoxic for sheep red blood cells coated with HLA-DRB1*0404 and type XI collagen peptides. These two observations have important pathological significance because they link directly an HLA susceptibility type to joint damage through the presence of anti-*Proteus mirabilis* antibodies causing damage to chondrocytes carrying HLA markers and to collagen XI present in hyaline cartilage.

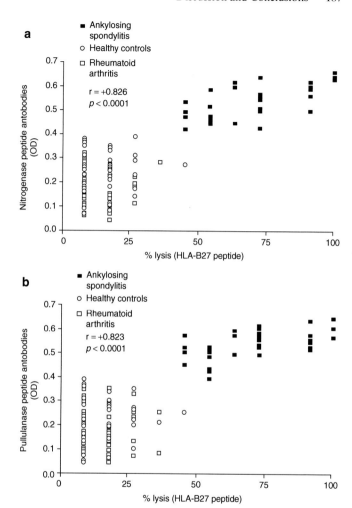

FIGURE 17.4 Correlation of anti-*Klebsiella* nitrogenase (**a**) and anti-*Klebsiella* pullulanase (**b**) IgG antibody levels for ankylosing spondylitis and rheumatoid arthritis patients and controls with percentage lysis of sheep *red* blood cells coated with HLA-B27 peptide (With kind permission from Wilson et al. (2003))

The pathological sequence could be summarised as follows:

'shared epitope' ▶ *Proteus* infection ▶ anti-*Proteus* antibodies ▶ joint damage

Similarly, ankylosing spondylitis patients have been shown to have increased levels of antibodies against synthetic peptides derived from *Klebsiella pneumoniae* and HLA-B*2705, and there was a significant correlation between anti-HLA-B*2705 antibodies and percentage lysis of sheep red cells coated with HLA-B*2705 peptide.

A similar situation is known to occur in rheumatic fever, where anti-*streptococcal* antibodies have been found to be cytotoxic for heart and fibroblast cell lines, because of molecular similarity between the *streptococcal* M protein and human cardiac myosin. (Cunningham et al. 1992).

The rheumatoid arthritis and ankylosing spondylitis patients used in our studies were deemed to be active in that their erythrocyte sedimentation rates were elevated. The high levels of *Proteus mirabilis* haemolysin, urease, HLA-DRB1*0404 and type XI collagen peptide antibodies were not due to nonspecific effects of inflammation because although ankylosing spondylitis patients were active, their levels of antibodies were similar to those found in healthy control subjects.

Antibodies against type XI collagen have been described in rheumatoid arthritis patients (Morgan et al. 1987). Furthermore, antibodies to type XI collagen have been found to be arthritogenic in DBA/1 mice (Boissier et al. 1990).

The α2 subunit of type XI collagen is a component of hyaline cartilage and is also present in non-cartilaginous tissue such as vitreous humour, which could be of relevance in episcleritis and scleromalacia perforans, conditions occurring in severe rheumatoid arthritis.

Proteus mirabilis haemolysin is a virulence factor contributing to the pathogenesis of the microorganism (Peerbooms et al. 1984).

The urease molecule of *Proteus mirabilis* facilitates infection of the kidneys and the urinary tract (Musher et al. 1975).

The haemolysin molecule from *Proteus mirabilis* has been shown to be a potent cytotoxic agent against renal proximal tubular epithelial cells, and some of the systemic and vascular manifestations of rheumatoid arthritis could occur as the result of the biological properties of this molecule (Mobley et al. 1991).

In conclusion, it would appear that cytotoxic properties of anti-*Proteus mirabilis* antibodies could be relevant in rheumatoid arthritis (Wilson et al. 2003).

References

Boissier MC, Chiochia G, Ronzière MC, Herbage D, Fournier C. Arthritogenicity of minor collagens (types IX and XI) in mice. Arthritis Rheum. 1990;33:1–9.

Cunningham MW, Antone SM, Gulizia JM, McManus BM, Fischetti VA, Gaunt CJ. Cytotoxic and viral neutralizing antibodies cross-react with streptococcal M protein, enteroviruses and human cardiac myosin. Proc Natl Acad Sci USA. 1992;89:1320–4.

Dybwad A, Forre O, Siuod M. Increased serum and synovial antibodies to immunoselected peptides in patients with rheumatoid arthritis. Ann Rheum Dis. 1996;55:437–41.

Fielder M, Pirt SJ, Tarpey I, Wilson C, Cunningham P, Ettelaie C, et al. Molecular mimicry and ankylosing spondylitis: possible role of a novel sequence in pullulanase of *Klebsiella pneumoniae*. FEBS Lett. 1995;369:243–8.

Mobley LTH, Chippendale GR, Swihart KG, Welch RA. Cytotoxicity of the Hpm A haemolysin and urease of *Proteus mirabilis, Proteus vulgaris*against cultured renal proximal tubular epithelial cells. Infect Immun. 1991;59:2036–42.

Morgan K, Clague RB, Collins I, Ayad S, Phinn SD, Holt PJL. Incidence of antibodies to native and denatured cartilage collagens (types II, IX and XI) and type I collagen in rheumatoid arthritis. Ann Rheum Dis. 1987;46:902–7.

Musher DM, Griffith DP, Yawn D, Rossen RD. The role of urease in pyelonephritis resulting in urinary tract infection with *Proteus*. J Infect Dis. 1975;31:177–81.

Newkirk MM, Goldbach-Mansky R, Senior BW, Klippel J, Schumacher HR, El-Gabalawy HS. Elevated levels of IgA and IgM antibodies to *Proteus mirabilis*and IgM antibodies to

*Escherichia coli*are associated with early rheumatoid factor (RF) positive rheumatoid arthritis. Rheumatology (Oxford). 2005;44:1433–41.

Peerbooms PGH, Marian A, Verweij JJ, MacLaren DM. Vero cell invasiveness of *Proteus mirabilis*. Infect Immun. 1984;43:1068–71.

Senior BW, McBride RDP, Morley KD, Kerr MA. The detection of raised levels of IgM to *Proteus mirabilis*in sera from patients with rheumatoid arthritis. J Med Microbiol. 1995;43:176–84.

Takeuchi F, Kosuge E, Matsuta K, Nakano K, Tokunaga K, Juji T et al. Antibody to a specific HLA-DRβ1 sequence in Japanese patients with rheumatoid arthritis. Arthritis Rheum. 1990;33:1867–8.

Wilson C, Rashid T, Tiwana H, Beyan H, Hughes L, Bansal S, et al. Cytotoxicity responses to peptide antigens in rheumatoid arthritis and ankylosing spondylitis. J Rheumatol. 2003;30:972–8.

Chapter 18
The Scientific Method of Sir Karl Popper

Contents

Sir Karl Popper, the Philosopher of Science

Sir Karl Popper was one of the most influential philosophers of science in the twentieth century and probably of all time. He proposed that a scientific theory could not be proved but could be disproved or falsified. He claimed that 'It must be possible for a scientific system to be refuted by experience. A theory that is not refutable by any conceivable event is non-scientific. Every "good" scientific theory is a prohibition: it

A. Ebringer, *Rheumatoid Arthritis and Proteus*,
DOI 10.1007/978-0-85729-950-5_18,
© Springer-Verlag London Limited 2012

forbids certain things to happen. The more a theory forbids, the better it is' (Popper 1963).

The theory that 'All tigers are carnivorous' is refuted or falsified by the observation of one vegetarian tiger.

The logical basis of scientific research is the method of bold conjectures and attempted refutations. The process can be described by the following oversimplified schema:

Problem ► Theory ► Experiment ► New Problem

His proposal that scientific studies should be based on rational analysis of existing theories and then submitted to severe tests by logical criticisms and experimental investigations is the basis of modern science.

A Biography of Karl Popper

The Austrian-British philosopher of science, Sir Karl Popper (1902–1994), was born in Vienna into a middle-class family. His father was a lawyer and his mother was a talented musician.

After the First World War, he attended the University of Vienna, reading mathematics, physics, psychology and physics. He graduated in 1928 and qualified as a secondary school teacher in mathematics.

In 1934, he published his first book, 'Logik der Forschung' (Logic of Scientific Research) a seminal study which established Popper's reputation as a philosopher (Popper 1959).

In December 1936, he accepted a lectureship at Canterbury College in Christchurch, New Zealand, and in January 1937, he and his wife left Austria for the Antipodes.

In New Zealand, he wrote 'The Poverty of Historicism' and the 2-volume 'The Open Society and its enemies'. He claimed these works were his contribution to the war effort. They were a powerful and critical, intellectual attack on totalitarian societies of both the Right and the Left. He stayed in New Zealand during the duration of the Second World War.

After the war, he obtained a Readership at the London School of Economics and Political Science. In the succeeding 23 years as Professor of Logic and Scientific Method, he had a worldwide impact in many fields from politics, science, philosophy, biology and sociology.

The Problem of Words and Their Meanings

In his autobiography 'The unended quest' Popper mentions a debate he had with his father about the Swedish dramatist Strindberg's autobiography where the writer was trying to extract the 'true' meanings of certain words. Popper continues:

> When I tried to press my objections that there was no such thing as a 'true' meaning, I was disturbed, indeed shocked that my father did not see the point. The issue seemed obvious to me. When we broke off, late at night I realized that I had failed to make much impact.
>
> There was a real gulf between us on an issue of importance. I tried strongly to impress on myself that I must always remember the principle of never arguing about words and their meanings.
>
> The quest for linguistic precision is analogous to the quest for certainty and both should be abandoned. It is always undesirable to make an effort to increase precision for its own sake since this leads to loss of clarity (Popper 1976).

It was the great merit of Popper to point out that 'science' starts with 'problems' and not with linguistic puzzles. It is the identification of the 'problem' that starts a research worker speculating as to how to arrive at a solution which will throw some light on the puzzle or question he is trying to answer. Without 'problems to resolve', without 'puzzles to elucidate' there is no science. Popper goes on to suggest that 'once we realize all scientific statements or hypotheses are guesses or conjectures and that the vast majority have turned to be eventually false, we can proceed to new ways of looking at scientific problems'.

In a famous passage, Karl Popper offers a way as how to handle this situation:

> Assume a young scientist meets a problem which he does not understand. What can he do? I suggest that even though he does not understand the problem, he can try to solve it and criticise his solution. Since he does not understand the problem, his solution will be a failure, a fact which will be brought out by criticism. In this way, a first step will be made towards pinpointing where the difficulty lies. This means precisely, that a first step will be made towards understanding the problem, for a problem is a difficulty and understanding a problem consists in finding out where the difficulty lies. And this can only be done by finding out why certain solutions do not work.
>
> So we learn to understand a problem by trying to solve it and by failing. When we have failed a hundred times, we may become even experts with respect to this particular problem. That is, if anybody proposes a solution we may see at once, whether there is any prospect of success for this proposal or the proposal will fail because of the difficulties which we know only too well from our own past failures (Popper 1972).

The question 'What kind of explanation may be satisfactory?' leads to the reply, 'An explanation in terms of testable theories and falsifiable universal laws and critical conditions'. An explanation of this kind will be the more satisfactory, the more highly testable these laws are thereby proceeding to better theories.

The Scientific Problem and Its Explanation

The aim of science is to find satisfactory explanations of whatever strikes us as being in need of an explanation. By explanation is meant a set of statements by which one describes the state of affairs to be explained, the 'explicandum'. The explanatory statement or 'explicans' is the object of our search and as a rule will not be known; thus, it will have to be discovered.

Thus a scientific explanation, the 'explicans', whenever it is a discovery will be the explanation of the known by the unknown.

The 'explicans', in order to be satisfactory must fulfil a number of conditions:

1. It must logically entail the 'explicandum', the problem.
2. The 'explicans' ought to be true, although in general it will not be known to be true. It must not be known to be false even after the most critical examination.
3. There must be independent evidence for the 'explicans'. In other words, it must be independent and avoid ad hoc or circular arguments.

   Consider the following dialogue:

   'Why is the sea so rough today ?'

   'Because Neptune is very angry'.

   'How doyou know Neptune is very angry ?'

   'Oh, don't you see how very rough the sea is !'

   The explanation is unsatisfactory because the only evidence for the 'explicans' is the 'explicandum', the problem itself.
4. In order that the 'explicans' should not be ad hoc, it must be rich in content. It must have a variety of testable consequences, which are different from the 'explicandum', the problem. It must lead to many 'Popper sequences' (Popper 1972).

Evolutionary Theory of Knowledge

On the 9th June 1989, Popper was asked to give his belated Inaugural Lecture at the London School of Economics (Popper 1999).

The title he chose was 'Towards an evolutionary theory of knowledge'. The lecture is relevant to all scientists or medical research workers who are grappling with problems involving studies in physics or biology. They are certainly relevant to the study of rheumatoid arthritis. He made the following points in describing the search for knowledge:

1. Knowledge has the character of expectations.
2. Expectations have usually the character of hypotheses, of conjectural or hypothetical knowledge: they are uncertain. And those who expect or who know may be quite unaware of this uncertainty.
3. Most kinds of knowledge are hypothetical or conjectural.

4. In spite of its uncertainty or its hypothetical character, much of our knowledge will be objectively true. It will correspond to the objective facts.

5. Therefore we must clearly distinguish between the truth of an expectation or a hypothesis and its certainty and therefore between the two ideas: the idea of truth and the idea of certainty.

6. There is much truth in our knowledge but little certainty. We must approach our hypotheses critically; we must test them as severely as we can, in order to find out whether they can be shown to be false after all.

7. Truth is objective: it is correspondence to the facts.

8. Certainty is rarely objective: it is usually no more than a feeling of trust, of conviction, although based on insufficient knowledge. Such feelings are dangerous since they are rarely well founded. They may turn us into hysterical fanatics who try to convince themselves of a certainty which they unconsciously know is not available.

9. The issue of social relativism is widely held, often by sociologists. Who study the ways of scientists and who think thereby they study science and scientific knowledge. Many of these sociologists do not believe in objective truth but think of truth as a sociological concept.

10. Some of them believe that truth is what the experts believe to be true. But in all science the experts are sometimes mistaken. Whenever there is a breakthrough, it means that the experts have been proved wrong. And that the facts, the objective facts were different from what the experts expected them to be.

11. It is our suppressed sense of our fallibility that is responsible for the despicable tendency to form cliques and go along with whatever seems to be fashionable. For I hold that science ought to strive for objective truth that depends only on the facts; on truth that is above human authority and above arbitration, and certainly above scientific fashions. Some sociologists fail to understand that this objectivity is a possibility towards which science should aim. Yet science has aimed at truth for at least for the last 2,500 years.

12. Philosophers and some scientists often assume that all our knowledge stems from our senses, from 'sense data' which our senses deliver. Some believe that the question: 'How do you know?' is in every case equivalent to the question 'What are the observations that entitle you to your assertion?' But seen from a biological point of view this kind of approach is a colossal mistake. For our senses tell us nothing without prior knowledge. This prior knowledge cannot in turn be the result of observation, it must be the result of evolution by trial and error as a solution or an attempt at a solution of a problem.

13. Observations or data may lead in science to the abandonment of a scientific theory and thereby induce some of us to think up a new tentative theory – a new trial. But the new theory is our product, our thought, our invention and a new theory is only rarely thought by more than a few people, even when there are many who agree on the refutation of the old theory. The few are those who see the new problem. Seeing a new problem may well be the most difficult step in creating a new theory (Popper 1999).

Bacon, Hume and Popper

Sir Francis Bacon (1561–1626) proposed that science consists of making observations about natural phenomena which then lead to theories. Repeatable observations lead to theories by the mechanism of 'induction'. David Hume (1711–1776) claimed that because B follows A, today, we cannot make the prediction that the same will happen tomorrow. In other words, Bacon's method of 'induction' does not exist. Thus, the assumption A causes B is based on mere habit or belief and this severely undermined the belief in empiricism and empirical observations. Bertrand Russell claimed that 'The growth of unreason and romantic philosophies in the nineteenth and twentieth centuries is a natural sequel to Hume's destruction of empiricism' (Russell 1946).

Popper was a great critic of the Baconian myth that all science starts with observations and then slowly and cautiously proceeds to theories. It was the great merit of Popper to point out that 'science' starts with 'problems'. It is the identification of the 'problem' that starts a research worker speculating as to how to arrive at a solution which will throw some light on the puzzle or question he is trying to answer. Without 'problems to resolve', without 'puzzles to elucidate' there is no science. Popper goes on to suggest that 'once we realize all scientific statements or hypotheses are guesses or conjectures and that the vast majority have turned out to be false, the Baconian myth becomes irrelevant'. This leads to the realization that attempts to find the truth are not final, but open to improvement; that knowledge is conjectural, that it consists of guesses or hypotheses rather than final and certain truths. Criticism and critical discussion with the help of experiments are our only means of getting nearer to the truth. It thus leads to the tradition of bold conjectures and free criticisms, the tradition which created the rational and scientific attitude of Western civilization.

Popper insisted that 'The task of science is the search for truth, that is for true theories. Yet it is not the only aim of science. We want more than mere truth, what we are looking is for interesting and "deep" truth which has a high degree of explanatory power. What we are looking for is answers to our problems'.

Popper's Scientific Method

The fundamental procedure of the growth of knowledge remains that of conjecture and refutation, of the elimination of unfit explanations.

A scientific result cannot be justified. It can only be criticised and tested.

Theories about how knowledge grows involve methods of trial and error.

Here is a tetradic scheme for the description of the growth of knowledge:

$$P(1) \blacktriangleright TT \blacktriangleright EE \blacktriangleright P(2)$$

Popper proposed a powerful analytical method to investigate scientific problems. The process can be described by the following simple schematic outline of how to tackle a scientific problem.

We start from a simple scientific 'problem 1'(P1) and try to solve it by a 'tentative theory' (TT1) which may or may not be correct. The theory will then be subjected to 'error elimination' (EE1) either by logical criticism or experimental studies. As a result of these investigations, a new fact will appear, 'problem 2' (P2) which in turn will require a scientific explanation. This is a 'Popper sequence'.

If each 'Popper sequence' generates new facts, then the original problem becomes richer in that it has more questions to resolve, but at the same time, the investigation gets closer to the truth of the inquiry, to the centre of the problem. The new facts uncovered by this 'Second Popper Sequence' are different from the 'First Sequence' because they are related to the logical properties of the hypothesis or 'tentative theory' and the facts that follow from the 'error elimination' steps.

The tetradic schema is an attempt to show that the results of criticism, of 'error elimination' (EE) applied to a 'tentative theory' (TT) leads as a rule to the emergence of a 'new problem' (P2).

Problems, after they have been solved and their solutions examined, tend to beget problem-children, new problems, often of greater depth and even greater fertility than the old ones (Popper 1972).

The best tentative theories, and all theories are tentative, are those which give rise to the deepest and unexpected results.

If the new problem (P2) turns out to be merely the old problem (P1) in disguise, then we say that one theory only manages to shift the problem.

The decisive point is, of course always, how well does one theory solve our original problem. At any rate, one of the things we wish to achieve is to learn something new.

The Hippocratic Oath, Popper and Medicine

The centre piece of the 'Hippocratic oath' states: '…The regimen I shall adopt for the benefit of the patients according to my ability and judgement and not for their hurt or for any wrong' (Singer and Underwood 1962).

Popperian analysis of a scientific problem, such as rheumatoid arthritis, may provide new clues or ideas for treatment. However, it is only when the therapeutic proposals arising from Popperian analysis are actually provided to the patients that will we know if the scientific problem has been solved.

If no therapeutic benefits accrue to the rheumatoid arthritis patients from anti-*Proteus* treatment, then the hypothesis that these microbes are involved in this disease will have been disproved and the question of the origin of this condition will have to await new and better theories.

References

Popper Karl R. The logic of scientific discovery. London: Hutchinson of London; 1959.

Popper Karl R. Conjectures and refutations. The growth of scientific knowledge. London: London Routledge and Kegan Paul; 1963.

Popper Karl R. Objective knowledge. An evolutionary approach. Oxford: Oxford University Press; 1972. p. 181.

Popper Karl R. Unended quest. An intellectual autobiography. London: Fontana; 1976.

Popper Karl R. Towards an evolutionary theory of knowledge. In: Karl Popper, editor. All life is problem solving. Oxon: Routledge; 1999. p. 57–73.

Russell B. History of western philosophy. London: George Allen & Unwin; 1946.

Singer C, Underwood EA. A short history of medicine. Oxford: Oxford Clarendon Press; 1962. p. 32.

Chapter 19
Rheumatoid Arthritis and 'Popper Sequences'

Contents

A. Ebringer, *Rheumatoid Arthritis and Proteus*,
DOI 10.1007/978-0-85729-950-5_19,
© Springer-Verlag London Limited 2012

Introduction to 'Popper Sequences'

The cause of rheumatoid arthritis has been investigated by the methods of Sir Karl Popper who claimed that a theory could not be proved by induction or any other methods but could be disproved.

A fact which was incompatible with a theory would thereby disprove it and this approach has provided a powerful new method to investigate scientific problems.

The 'Popper sequences' consist of four stages:

First is the 'scientific problem' (P1 = Problem).

Secondly is the attempted solution or 'theory' (TT = Tentative Theory).

Thirdly is the attempted falsification of the theory by 'experiments or observations' (EE = Error Elimination).

Finally there is the generation of new knowledge which creates 'new problems' and 'new facts' (P2 = New problem).

Preliminary investigations have shown that 'Popper sequences' provide new ways of looking at scientific problems such as rheumatoid arthritis or ankylosing spondylitis.

If the cause of rheumatoid arthritis can be found, then appropriate steps could be taken in the early stages of the condition so that both medical problems of the patients and financial costs to society can be minimised to the mutual benefits of both groups.

Components of a 'Popper Sequence'

The sequence of a 'Popper Sequence' could be summarised as follows:

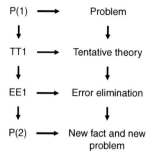

The second problem (P2) is different from the first; it is the result of the new situation that has arisen because of the tentative theories (TT1) and the error elimination (EE1) which consist of logical analysis or criticism and experimental investigations suggested by the 'Tentative theories' (TT1).

First Popper Sequence

The link between rheumatoid arthritis and human histocompatibility antigens, particularly HLA-DW4, was discovered by Stastny in 1976, using leucocyte cultures obtained from American rheumatoid arthritis patients.

Later this link between class II HLA antigens was confirmed when HLA-DR4 was demonstrated in English rheumatoid arthritis patients to be present more frequently than in the general population.

American research workers have identified that the common denominator in these HLA sequences from positions 70 to 74, encoding amino acids Gln-Arg-Arg-Ala-Ala (QRRAA) specific for HLA-DR1, HLA-DR4 (DW14 and DW15), was found to occur in RA patients.

The sequence of this region closely resembles the one in HLA-DR4 (DW4), there being only one amino acid substitution at position 71 from arginine to lysine. However, this is a conservative substitution since both arginine and lysine are positively charged amino acids. Glutamic acid (E) at position 69 is common to all DR-β1 molecules.

Therefore, the hexameric sequence EQR(K)RAA between amino acid positions 69 and 74 forms a powerful antigenic determinant. This hexameric sequence forms the basis of the 'shared epitope' (SE) which is found in some 90% of RA patients whilst the combined frequency of these genes in the general population is about 35%.

There are two ways of explaining this observation: either HLA-DR1/4 molecules present some antigens to immune cells or the EQR(K)RAA sequence resembles or shows 'molecular mimicry' to some component of bacteria or viruses present in the environment. Since 'molecular mimicry' appeared to work in rheumatic fever and Sydenham's chorea, we chose this approach to study the rheumatoid arthritis problem.

This leads to the first Popper sequence:

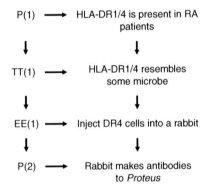

The result of the 'First Popper sequence' suggests that *Proteus* bacteria are somehow linked to HLA-DR4. This raises the new problem (P2) that *Proteus* bacteria may be involved in the onset or origin of rheumatoid arthritis.

However, we are not sure whether this is a property of HLA-DR4 lymphocytes or the rabbit may have been inadvertently immunised or exposed to *Proteus* bacteria whilst in the animal house.

Therefore, this observation must be checked against tissue typing sera and this leads to the Second Popper sequence.

Second Popper Sequence

It is possible that the rabbit exhibiting anti-*Proteus* antibodies following immunisation with HLA-DR4 lymphocytes may have been infected in the cage. Therefore, the fortuitous observation of anti-*Proteus* antibodies could be an artefact.

It was considered that to establish that *Proteus* microorganisms were somehow related to rheumatoid arthritis, they had to be linked to the HLA-DR4 specificity by more reliable methods than xenogeneic rabbit immunisation.

The first clear demonstration of cross-reactivity between HLA-B27 and *Klebsiella* occurred when allogeneic anti-HLA-B27 tissue typing sera bound to *Klebsiella* antigens to a greater extent than HLA tissue typing sera specific for other HLA antigens (Avakian et al. 1980).

A similar approach was adopted to study this problem. Following an initial pilot study, 12 anti-DR4 tissue typing sera and 17 non-DR4 tissue typing sera (anti-DR1, DR2, DR3, DR7, DR11 and DR52) (Courtesy of Dr. Julie Awad, London Hospital) were tested under code, by ELISA for their capacity to bind to *Proteus mirabilis* and *Escherichia coli* microorganisms.

Anti-DR4 tissue typing sera were found to bind to *Proteus* to a significantly greater extent ($p < 0.001$) whilst no such increased binding was observed with *Escherichia coli* microorganisms (Fig. 19.1) (Ebringer et al. 1988).

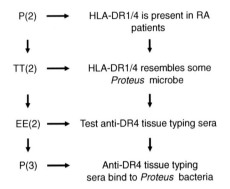

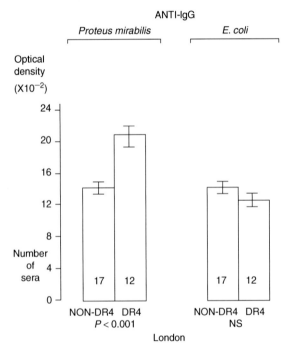

FIGURE 19.1 Antibody binding (mean ± standard error) OD units by HLA-DR tissue typing sera measured by ELISA against *Proteus mirabilis* and *Escherichia coli* bacteria (With permission from Ebringer et al. (1988))

It is interesting to note that rheumatoid arthritis occurs 3–4-times more frequently in women than in men, and the suggestion that *Proteus* bacteria might be involved immediately raises the idea that an upper urinary tract infection might cause the onset of the disease.

The microbe *E. coli* accounts for about 70–80% of urinary tract infections in women, and these usually involve or cause cystitis in the bladder. This microbe did not appear during the rabbit immunisation with HLA-DR4 lymphocytes.

Another 10–15% are due to infections by *Proteus* in the upper urinary tract.

Other bacteria, such as *Klebsiella*, account for the remainder of urinary tract infections.

The possibility arises that rheumatoid arthritis patients may have been infected by *Proteus* bacteria which are responsible for the second commonest cause of urinary tract infections.

This forms the basis of the 'Third Popper sequence'.

Third Popper Sequence

Antibodies to *Proteus* bacteria may be present in rheumatoid arthritis patients.

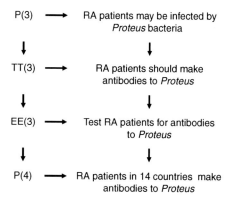

P(3) ⟶ RA patients may be infected by *Proteus* bacteria

TT(3) ⟶ RA patients should make antibodies to *Proteus*

EE(3) ⟶ Test RA patients for antibodies to *Proteus*

P(4) ⟶ RA patients in 14 countries make antibodies to *Proteus*

Antibodies to *Proteus* bacteria were first reported from England in 1985 and subsequently from many different countries.

The list of countries and the year of publication of the presence of elevated levels of anti-*Proteus* antibodies is as follows:

	Country	Year of study
1.	England	1985
2.	Ireland	1988
3.	France	1994
4.	Scotland	1995
5.	Norway	1995
6.	Bermuda	1995
7.	Japan	1997
8.	India	1997
9.	Netherlands	1998
10.	Spain	1999
11.	Russia	2000
12.	Finland	2004
13.	USA	2005
14.	Canada	2005

The list of the 24 towns throughout the world from where elevated levels of antibodies to *Proteus* have been reported is as follows:

UK	London
	Stevenage
	Winchester
	Newcastle
	Glasgow
	Edinburgh
	Dundee

France	Brest
	Toulouse
Ireland	Dublin
Spain	Barcelona
Norway	Oslo
Japan	Otsu
	Tokyo
Bermuda	Hamilton
Netherlands	Amsterdam
Finland	Helsinki
India	Delhi
Russia	Moscow
Slovakia	Pieštany
USA	Philadelphia
	Washington
Canada	Montreal
	Winnipeg

The question arises whether these antibodies to *Proteus* are specific to rheumatoid arthritis patients or could they occur in other chronic diseases and this brings us to the 'Fourth Popper sequence'.

Fourth Popper Sequence

An examination of antibodies against *Proteus* in the serum of active rheumatoid arthritis patients was compared to patients with other chronic diseases, such as ankylosing spondylitis, uveitis, sarcoidosis, Crohn's disease (Tiwana et al. 1997), systemic lupus erythematosus and ulcerative colitis.

Clearly acute infections involving these microbes may have elevated levels of anti-*Proteus* antibodies, but we are concerned only with chronic diseases involving many systems.

There was no elevation in antibodies against *Proteus* bacteria in these other chronic diseases.

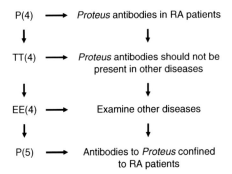

The next problem arises as to the site where these bacteria are located.

This brings us to the 'Fifth Popper sequence'.

Fifth Popper Sequence

The location of the *Proteus* bacteria in active RA patients has so far not been resolved:

> Are these bacteria to be found in the respiratory tract, the gastro-intestinal tract or the urinary tract?
> It is possible that the upper urinary tract is the site of the *Proteus* infection.

In a survey of 89 rheumatoid arthritis patients, *Proteus mirabilis* was isolated from the urine of 63% (47/75) female ($p<0.001$) and 50% (7/14) male patients compared to a frequency of isolation in healthy women of 32% (38/119) and 11% (13/115) in men.

Non-rheumatoid arthritis patients were those with osteoarthritis, gout or psoriasis, and their urine samples showed similar results as those observed in healthy controls.

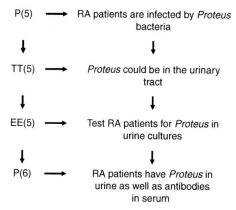

P(5) ⟶ RA patients are infected by *Proteus* bacteria

TT(5) ⟶ *Proteus* could be in the urinary tract

EE(5) ⟶ Test RA patients for *Proteus* in urine cultures

P(6) ⟶ RA patients have *Proteus* in urine as well as antibodies in serum

There appears to be a correlation between positive urine cultures for *Proteus* in active rheumatoid arthritis patients when they have at the same time, elevated levels of antibodies against *Proteus* bacteria.

These five 'Popper sequences' have identified so far that HLA-DR1/4 resembles *Proteus*; antibodies to this microbe are present in RA patients, no such antibodies are present in other chronic diseases and the site of infection would appear to be the urinary tract.

This brings us to the next 'Popper sequence' whether *Proteus* is the only microbe present in rheumatoid arthritis patients or could antibodies be detected against other microbiological agents.

Sixth Popper Sequence

Many studies have been carried out by different independent groups on antibodies against various microbial antigens in patients with rheumatoid arthritis.

The high titre of anti-*Proteus* antibodies would appear to be specific because there was no such elevation in antibodies against 27 other microbial agents (Table 19.1) (Rashid and Ebringer 2007a).

Table 19.1 Statistical values of antibodies against various microbial species in patients with rheumatoid arthritis

Reference	Proteus	Klebsiella	Esch.	Yersinia	Salm.	Chlam.	Shigella	Pseud.	Serratia	Campyl.	NBF spp.	Viruses
Ebringer et al. (1985)	<0.001	NS										NS(4)[a]
Khalafpour et al. (1988)	<0.05	NS										
Deighton et al. (1992)	<0.001											
Subair et al. (1995)	<0.001		NS							NS(3)		
Fielder et al. (1995)	<0.001		NS		NS							
Tiwana et al. (1996)	<0.001		NS					NS	NS			
Tiwana et al. (1997)	<0.001	NS	NS							NS(10)		
Tani et al. (1997)	<0.001	NS	NS									

Study						
Wanchu et al. (1997)	<0.001		NS			
Blankenberg-Sprenkels et al. (1998)	<0.001	NS				NS
Newkirk et al. (2005)	<0.001	<0.05	NS	NS	NS	NS
Rashid et al. (2004)	<0.001	NS				NS

NS not significant, *Esch Escherichia coli*, *Salm Salmonella*, Chlam *Chlamydia*, Pseud *Pseudomonas*, Campyl *Campylobacter*, *NBF* normal bowel flora

The "p" values compare patients to controls

[a]Number of microbes tested

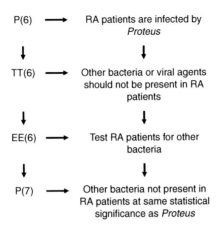

The majority of these studies showed that anti-*Proteus* antibodies were present in rheumatoid arthritis patients at a statistically significant level ($p < 0.001$) in 11 out of 12 studies and once, at a lower level of significance ($p < 0.05$). In one study, anti-*Escherichia coli* antibodies were slightly elevated ($p < 0.05$), but at the same time, the anti-*Proteus* titre was clearly significantly elevated ($p < 0.001$) in the rheumatoid arthritis patients. It appears that *Proteus* bacteria are clearly involved in rheumatoid arthritis patients, but the pathological mechanism of joint damage and its link to HLA require further examination. We still do not know which component of HLA-DR1/4 is associated with *Proteus* bacteria.

This brings us to the 'Seventh Popper sequence'.

Seventh Popper Sequence

The 'shared epitope' or SE is the main amino acid sequence of HLA-DR1/4 molecules associated with an increased susceptibility to develop rheumatoid arthritis.

However, it is not clear whether EQR(K)RAA is somehow linked to *Proteus* bacteria.

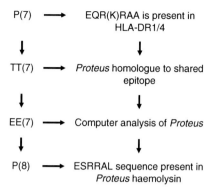

P(7) ⟶ EQR(K)RAA is present in HLA-DR1/4

TT(7) ⟶ *Proteus* homologue to shared epitope

EE(7) ⟶ Computer analysis of *Proteus*

P(8) ⟶ ESRRAL sequence present in *Proteus* haemolysin

The 'error elimination' (EE7) in this Popper sequence consists of carrying out a computer analysis of the components of the *Proteus* bacteria to see if they resemble or show 'molecular mimicry' to the EQR(K)RAA sequence.

Computer analysis shows that there is a sequence in *Proteus* haemolysin from amino acid positions 32–36 (ESRRAL) which is almost identical in shape to the EQR(K)RAA sequence of the 'shared epitope' found in HLA-DR1/4 molecules. Thus, the presence of antibodies to *Proteus* bacteria may also contain antibodies to *Proteus* haemolysin. Such antibodies could bind to the EQRRAA sequences found in HLA-DR1/4 molecules and following complement activation causes inflammation with consequent tissue damage.

A clinical feature of rheumatoid arthritis, as opposed to ankylosing spondylitis, is that it affects predominantly the small joints of the hands and feet and this leads to the next Popper sequence.

Eighth Popper Sequence

The majority of urinary tract infections are caused by *Escherichia coli* which usually produces cystitis in the bladder. However, rheumatoid arthritis patients do not have antibodies to this microbe.

A chief distinguishing feature between the urinary bacteria *Escherichia coli* and *Proteus mirabilis* is the presence of the enzyme urease. *Proteus* bacteria are positive for urease whilst *Escherichia coli* microbes are negative for urease, and the presence of this enzyme is used in distinguishing these bacteria in urine cultures.

The question arises whether urease may show 'molecular mimicry' or molecular similarity to some collagens found preferentially in small joints.

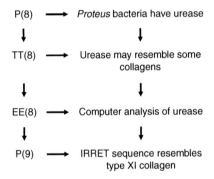

The IRRET sequence of *Proteus* urease from amino acid positions 337–341 is almost identical in shape or shows molecular mimicry with an α-2 (XI) collagen sequence LRREI from amino acid positions 421–425.

Type XI collagen is found predominantly in hyaline cartilage which is present in the joints of both hands and feet. Furthermore, rheumatoid arthritis patients have antibodies to *Proteus* urease and also to sequences not known to cross-react with self-antigens, thereby indicating that a *Proteus* infection has occurred (Rashid et al. 2007b).

Ninth Popper Sequence

Rheumatoid arthritis is characterised by inflammatory episodes, and their occurrence can be monitored by the presence of an elevated erythrocyte sedimentation rate (ESR) and/or elevated C-reactive protein level (CRP).

It is important here to distinguish between clinical assessments of pain as measured by subjective 'analogue scales' whereby the patient indicates on a scale of 1–10 the degree of discomfort and pain felt, as opposed to an objective measurement of inflammation as given by ESR or CRP levels. The usual level which determines active disease and presence of biochemical inflammation is an ESR > 30 mm/h or a C-reactive protein level > 15 mg/l.

The crucial issue is whether such inflammatory episodes could be triggered by the high titres of anti-*Proteus* antibodies that have been identified in rheumatoid arthritis patients.

The Popperian question or proposal arises whether such cytopathic effects can be demonstrated as an indication that anti-*Proteus* antibodies are the first triggers or agents in this disease.

This will provide an answer to the important question 'Do rheumatoid arthritis sera produce or cause tissue damage?'

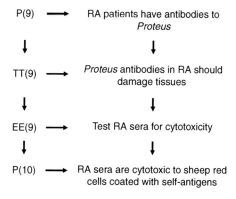

P(9) ⟶ RA patients have antibodies to *Proteus*

TT(9) ⟶ *Proteus* antibodies in RA should damage tissues

EE(9) ⟶ Test RA sera for cytotoxicity

P(10) ⟶ RA sera are cytotoxic to sheep red cells coated with self-antigens

Sera from active rheumatoid arthritis patients were tested by a complement-mediated cytotoxicity assay.

Sheep red cells were coated with EQRRAA (HLA-DR1/4) or ESRRAL (*Proteus* haemolysin) peptides and compared to sera from patients with ankylosing spondylitis and healthy blood donors.

Rheumatoid arthritis sera had cytotoxic activity to both EQRRAA- or ESRRAL-coated peptides, thereby suggesting that these were the initiating or trigger factors in the onset of disease. However, sheep red cells coated with EDERAA peptide, an HLA group which is not linked to the occurrence of rheumatoid arthritis, were found not to react with the rheumatoid arthritis sera.

Similar cytotoxic results were obtained when sheep red cells were coated with either IRRET (*Proteus* urease) or LRREI (type XI collagen) peptides and tested with rheumatoid arthritis sera.

It has been suggested that cytotoxic and inflammatory activity in joint tissues leads to denaturation of connective tissue components such as filaggrin which may produce 'cyclical citrullinated proteins' (CCP) and these in turn will evoke anti-CCP antibodies. This brings us to the next Popper sequence.

Tenth Popper Sequence

Anti-CCP antibodies have been demonstrated to be present in many cases of rheumatoid arthritis, several years before the appearance of clinical symptoms of the disease (Avouac et al. 2006).

The main component of these antigens is citrulline which is derived from the positively charged amino acid arginine. Tissue components that contain arginine when denatured by peptidyl arginine deiminase (PAD) will lead to the formation of citrulline-containing compounds. Peptidyl arginine deiminase (PAD) is an enzyme present in inflammatory cells, such as polymorphs, especially neutrophils and macrophages (Schellekens et al. 1998).

It is pertinent to note that both *Proteus* cross-reacting peptides, ESRRAL and IRRET, contain each an arginine doublet which could be acted on by peptidyl arginine deiminase (PAD) enzymes from granulocytes to form cyclical citrullinated proteins (CCP).

Similarly, the 'shared epitope' EQRRAA and the type XI sequence LRREI cross-reacting with a sequence in *Proteus* urease, also each have an arginine doublet which could be acted on by PAD enzymes to produce CCP.

There are thus four different molecules involved in rheumatoid arthritis where each one contains an 'arginine doublet'.

Whether the polyclonal response of anti-CCP antibodies found in rheumatoid arthritis patients is involved with these arginine-containing peptide sequences awaits further examination.

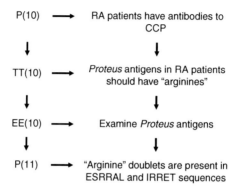

The presence of inflammation in joints with consequent tissue damage raises the question that HLA antigens and collagens may be denatured and lead to the formation of autoantibodies. Such autoantibodies could then be detected by bacterial cross-reactive antigens such as ESRRAL found in *Proteus* haemolysin or the IRRET sequence found in *Proteus* urease.

This question brings us to the next Popper sequence.

Eleventh Popper Sequence

If *Proteus* bacteria have infected rheumatoid arthritis patients, then antibodies to both cross-reacting (HLA-DR1/4 and type XI collagen) and non cross-reacting antigens should be demonstrable in such patients.

Computer analysis of *Proteus* urease led to the discovery of a sequence which was highly antigenic (KELRQEER)

(Positions 85–99) since it had several charged amino acids but proteonomic analysis could not identify any similarity or cross-reactivity to human self-antigens.

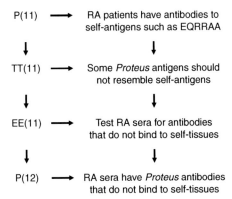

ELISA analysis was carried out to determine whether antibodies to this sequence (KELRQEER) were present in 60 active rheumatoid arthritis patients. Significantly elevated levels of antibodies ($p < 0.001$) were found to KELRQEER as well as to the sequences ESRRAL found in *Proteus* haemolysin cross-reacting with HLA-DR1/4 and IRRET sequence found in *Proteus* urease cross-reacting with type XI collagen when compared to healthy blood donors (Rashid et al. 2007b).

This is compelling evidence that active rheumatoid arthritis patients have been exposed and infected by *Proteus* bacteria.

Twelfth Popper Sequence

It would appear that rheumatoid arthritis is caused by an upper urinary tract infection by *Proteus* bacteria (Fig. 19.2).

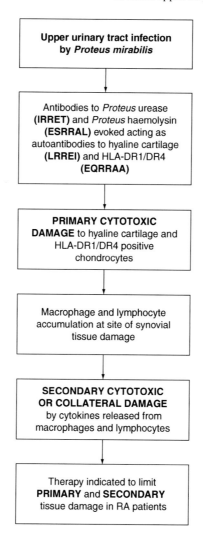

FIGURE 19.2 Proposed pathogenesis of rheumatoid arthritis following an upper urinary tract infection by *Proteus* bacteria

There are two phases to the development of this disease:

Firstly, there is 'primary damage' which is due an infection in the upper urinary tract by *Proteus* bacteria and this leads to the formation of anti-*Proteus* antibodies in the local lymph nodes. One of these anti-*Proteus* antibodies has an anti-collagen XI specificity and, therefore, a cytotoxic activity directed against the hyaline cartilage found in the joints. This is the link between the microbe and the joint. Another anti-*Proteus* antibody has an anti-haemolysin activity which targets cells bearing the 'shared epitope' namely chondrocytes expressing HLA-DR1 and HLA-DR4 antigens. When elevated levels of anti-*Proteus* antibodies are present and with complement activation, there will be cytotoxic and inflammatory damage in joints which carry hyaline cartilage.

Secondly, there is 'secondary damage' due to the development of nonspecific tissue damage in the joints which leads to inflammation and accumulation of inflammatory cells, T and B lymphocytes, interleukins, tumour necrosis factors and numerous degradative enzymes associated with inflammation which then cause 'secondary damage'. The antitumour necrosis factor biologicals are effective in reducing this 'secondary damage' due to the ongoing process of inflammation started by the anti-*Proteus* inflammation.

However, the disease could also be controlled by reducing the first phase, the 'primary damage', the one associated with the *Proteus* infection which leads to the production of these damaging cytotoxic autoantibodies and which are the first agents causing joint damage.

The 'primary damage' also involves preferentially attacking the individuals bearing the susceptibility HLA antigens, enshrined in the 'shared epitope'.

This leads to the next Popper sequence.

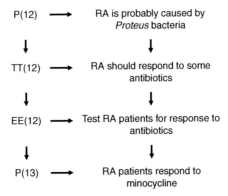

P(12) ⟶ RA is probably caused by *Proteus* bacteria

↓   ↓

TT(12) ⟶ RA should respond to some antibiotics

↓   ↓

EE(12) ⟶ Test RA patients for response to antibiotics

↓   ↓

P(13) ⟶ RA patients respond to minocycline

The use of minocycline, initially advocated by Thomas MacPherson Brown, has been found to be effective in several controlled studies (O'Dell et al. 1999).

However, minocycline is a bacteriostatic agent and probably not the most effective antibiotic against *Proteus* bacteria.

The use of nitrofurantoin or quinolone antibiotics, such as nalidixic acid, norfloxacin, ciprofloxacine, ofloxacin or levofloxacine, should be evaluated in the treatment of rheumatoid arthritis.

Discussion and Conclusion

The probable cause of the onset of rheumatoid arthritis has been identified through the demonstration of 12 'Popper sequences', each of which provided a new fact about the disease. If any other theory were to be suggested, it would have to account for the 'new facts' uncovered by this Popperian analysis.

The accessory properties of the rheumatoid arthritis problem, such as the link to smokers, could be explained by the published evidence that smokers have a greater frequency of urinary tract infections. Onset after pregnancy would appear also to be associated again with urinary tract infections (Nymand 1974).

These conclusions involving numerous experimental results open a new approach to the treatment of this crippling, arthritic disease by using anti-*Proteus* therapy together with existing modalities of treatment. Any new theory proposed for the causation of rheumatoid arthritis must also explain the 'new facts' uncovered by these 12 'Popper sequences' (Ebringer et al. 2010).

In science, we are trying to get closer to the truth, but in medicine, the results of our investigations should help the patient as suggested by the Hippocratic oath.

Current therapy of rheumatoid arthritis involves the use of agents such as methotrexate and anti-TNF biologicals which significantly reduce the degree of inflammation (Zintzaras et al. 2008). However, biological therapy is associated with an increased risk of skin cancers (Wolfe and Michaud 2007). The discovery that rheumatoid arthritis is triggered or caused by a *Proteus* urinary tract infection opens a new approach to the treatment of this disabling arthritic disease.

In future, treatment of rheumatoid arthritis will involve not only the use of established modalities of therapy, such as methotrexate and anti-TNF biologicals, (Vital and Emery 2008) but also a protocol involving anti-urinary tract infection management consisting of specific antibiotics, high fluid intake and even the use of dietary agents such as cranberry juice which have been found useful in treating urinary tract infections (Avorn et al. 1994).

The discovery that a urinary tract infection is involved in the onset of rheumatoid arthritis would tend to indicate that there will be more patients developing this disease in the future. As there is a worldwide trend in an increasing life expectancy, the greater incidence of urinary tract infections in an ageing population, especially among women, will inevitably lead to a greater number of patients suffering from this disabling, arthritic disease.

The identification of *Proteus* as the causative agent may lead to a greater likelihood of diagnosing this disease in its early stages, especially before X-ray changes have occurred with its irreversible joint and bony complications.

The role of anti-*Proteus* therapy in the management of rheumatoid arthritis requires an evaluation by multi-centre studies (Ebringer et al. 2003).

References

Avakian H, Welsh J, Ebringer A, Entwistle CC. Ankylosing spondylitis, HLA-B27 and *Klebsiella*. II. Cross-reactivity studies with human tissue typing sera. Br J Exp Pathol. 1980;61:92–6.

Avorn J, Monane M, Gurwitz JH, Glynn RJ, Chodnovskiy I, Lipsitz LA. Reduction of bacteriuria and pyuria after ingestion of cranberry juice. JAMA. 1994;271:751–4.

Avouac J, Gossec L, Dougados M. Diagnostic and predictive value of anti-cyclic citrullinated protein antibodies in rheumatoid arthritis: a systematic, literature review. Ann Rheum Dis. 2006;65:845–51.

Blankenberg-Sprenkels SHD, Fielder M, Feldkamp TEW, Tiwana H, Wilson C, Ebringer A. Antibodies to *Klebsiella pneumoniae* in Dutch patients with ankylosing spondylitis and acute anterior uveitis and to *Proteus mirabilis* in rheumatoid arthritis. J Rheumatol. 1998;25:743–7.

Deighton CM, Gray SW, Biant AJ, Walker DJ. Specificity of the *Proteus* antibody response in rheumatoid arthritis. Ann Rheum Dis. 1992;51:1206–7.

Ebringer A, Ptaszynska T, Corbett M, Wilson C, Macafee Y, Avakian H, et al. Antibodies to *Proteus* in rheumatoid arthritis. Lancet. 1985;2:305–7.

Ebringer A, Cox NL, Abuljadayel I, Ghuloom M, Khalafpour S, Ptaszynska T, et al. *Klebsiella* antibodies in ankylosing spondylitis and *Proteus* antibodies in rheumatoid arthritis. Br J Rheumatol. 1988;27(Suppl II):72–85.

Ebringer A, Rashid T, Wilson C. Rheumatoid arthritis: proposal for the early use of anti-bacterial therapy. Scand J Rheumatol. 2003;32:2–11.

Ebringer A, Rashid T, Wilson C. Rheumatoid arthritis, *Proteus*, anti-CCP antibodies and Karl Popper. Autoimmun Rev. 2010;9:216–23.

Fielder M, Tiwana H, Youinou P, Le Goff P, Deonarian R, Wilson C, et al. The specificity of the anti-*Proteus* antibody response in tissue-typed rheumatoid arthritis (RA) patients from Brest. Rheumatol Int. 1995;15:79–82.

Khalafpour S, Ebringer A, Abuljadayel I, Corbett M. Antibodies to *Klebsiella* and *Proteus* microrganisms in ankylosing spondylitis and rheumatoid arthritis patients measured by ELISA. Br J Rheumatol. 1988;27(Suppl II):86–9.

Newkirk MM, Goldbach-Mansky R, Senior BW, Klippel J, Schumacher Jr HR, El-Gabalawy HS. Elevated levels of IgM and IgA antibodies to *Proteus mirabilis* and IgM antibodies to *Escherichia coli* are associated with early rheumatoid factor (RF)-positive rheumatoid arthritis. Rheumatology. 2005;44:1433–41.

Nymand G. Maternal smoking and immunity. Lancet. 1974;2:1379–80.

O'Dell JR, Paulsen G, Haire CE, Blakely K, Palmer W, Wees S, et al. Treatment of early seropositive rheumatoid arthritis with minocycline. Arthritis Rheum. 1999;42:1691–5.

Rashid T, Ebringer A. Rheumatoid arthritis is linked to *Proteus* – the evidence. Clin Rheumatol. 2007a;26:1036–43.

Rashid T, Jayakumar KS, Binder A, Ellis S, Cunningham P, Ebringer A. Rheumatoid arthritis patients have elevated antibodies to cross-reactive and non-cross reactive antigens from *Proteus* microbes. Clin Exp Rheumatol. 2007b;25:259–67.

Rashid T, Leirisalo-Repo M, Tani Y, Hukuda S, Kobayashi S, Wilson C, et al. Antibacterial and antipeptide antibodies in Japanese and Finnish patients with rheumatoid arthritis. Clin Rheumatol. 2004;23:134–41.

Schellekens GA, de Jong BA, Van den Hoogen FH, Van de Putte LB, van Venrooij WJ. Citrulline is an essential constituent of antigenic determinants recognized by rheumatoid arthritis specific auto-antibodies. J Clin Invest. 1998;101:273–81.

Subair H, Tiwana H, Fielder M, Binder A, Cunningham K, Ebringer A, et al. Elevation in anti-*Proteus* antibodies in patients with rheumatoid arthritis from Bermuda and England. J Rheumatol. 1995;22:1825–8.

Tani Y, Tiwana H, Hukuda S, Nishioka J, Fielder M, Wilson C, et al. Antibodies to *Klebsiella*, *Proteus* and HLA-B27 peptides in Japanese patients with ankylosing spondylitis and rheumatoid arthritis. J Rheumatol. 1997;24:109–14.

Tiwana H, Wilson C, Cunningham P, Binder A, Ebringer A. Antibodies to four gram-negative bacteria in rheumatoid arthritis which share sequences with the rheumatoid arthritis susceptibility motif. Br J Rheumatol. 1996;35:592–4.

Tiwana H, Wilson C, Walmsley RS, Wakefield AJ, Smith MSN, Cox NL, et al. Antibody responses to gut bacteria in ankylosing spondylitis, rheumatoid arthritis, Crohn's disease and ulcerative colitis. Rheumatol Int. 1997;17:11–6.

Vital EM, Emery P. The development of targeted therapies in rheumatoid arthritis. J Autoimmun. 2008;31:219–27.

Wanchu A, Deodhar SD, Sharma M, Gupta V, Bambery P, Sud A. Elevated levels of anti-*Proteus* antibodies in patients with active rheumatoid arthritis. Indian J Med Res. 1997;105:39–42.

Wolfe F, Michaud K. Biologic treatment of rheumatoid arthritis and the risk of malignancy. Arthritis Rheum. 2007;56:2886–95.

Zintzaras E, Dahabreh LJ, Giannouli S, Voulgarelis M, Moutsopoulos HM. Infliximab and methotrexate in the treatment of rheumatoid arthritis: a systematic review and meta-analysis of dosage regimens. Clin Ther. 2008;30:1939–55.

Index

A. Ebringer, *Rheumatoid Arthritis and Proteus,*
DOI 10.1007/978-0-85729-950-5,
© Springer-Verlag London Limited 2012